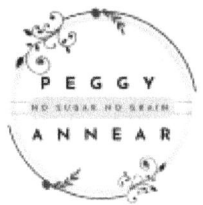

No Sugar No Grain
Roadmap to Quit Sugars
The Low Carb No Sugar Solution

by Peg E. Annear
2024 © All Rights Reserved
ISBN 9781763626508

Table of Contents

Our Sugar Addiction Problem 1
How Does Blood Sugar Work? 5
Are Carbs and Sugars Equal? 9
What is a Detox Diet? 11
How Snacking Effects Insulin 16
How Artificial Sweeteners Differ 17
GI Spikes and Fructose 19
How Controlling Insulin Levels Boosts Fat Loss 25
The Exercise Myth; You've Been Lied to...Here's the Truth 27
Preparing for the 7 Day Elimination Plan 31
How to Read Food Labels for Weight Loss 33
What is an Acceptable Amount of Carbohydrates? 35
Foods to Eat for Energy & Success 39
6 Top Sugar Free Beverages 41
How Fats Stabilize Sugar Cravings 44
Cream vs Milk - Surprising Facts 46
Foods to Avoid for Sustained Success 49
Detailed Vegetable List by Ranking 53
Sugar Smart Tips to Achieve Your Goals 59
How to Quit Sugar & Beat Cravings 69
The Low Sugar Low Fat Myth 74
Complex Carb Count in Common Foods 79
Total Carbs or Net Carbs? 80
How to Control Carb Detox Side Effects 81
7 Day Low Carb Meals (No Calorie Counting) 84
Day 1 91
Day 2 102
Day 3 113
Day 4 128
Day 5 140
Day 6 150
Day 7 162
Research & Resources 176

Download Planner & Organizer from the Author 177

Introduction

We all stumble at times, but you're simply awesome for tackling sugar addiction.

I'll guide you through step-by-step and show you how to take control.

Now you can finally feel and look amazing. Here's to celebrating a healthier happier you!

****

→ This book is filled with **guidance and tools to achieve your goals.**

→ You will be mentored through a complete understanding of **how sugar and carbs affect your body & how to beat the cravings.**

→ **Uncover obstacles** and learn how to steer clear of them.

→ Get ready for some surprising insights about sugar, carbs and your body.

→ NO need to count Calories!

→ **Find a new you.**

Starting here...

Inside This Book

*Discover the often unknown secrets of sugar and carbohydrates, and master the tricks to understanding and controlling your body's reactions for positive change.

*Transform your life with 7 days of delicious, easy-to-make, no sugar, keto and diabetic friendly low-carb recipes, totaling 38 delectable options.

*Gain insight into Nutritional breakdown in total carbs, sugars, protein, fiber, fats & calories.

*Be armed with knowledge that explains how to identify hidden sugars and minimize insulin spikes to aid your fat burning weight loss goals.

*Each recipe is presented in an easy-to-read format with notes and plenty of optional ingredients, offering flexibility to fit into your busy lifestyle.

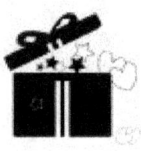

Bonus Gifts (PDF Downloads via QR code / link)
★ Detailed Weekly Meal Planner
★ Shopping List Planner & Organizer

About the Author

Hi, I'm Peggy. After a decade of struggling with my weight and inflammatory issues, I found the Paleo diet and began cutting out sugar in 2018. A low carb diet changed my relationship with food and led to a 15 kg weight loss along with better health and energy.

My passions include researching holistic health, cooking, writing and graphic design. Fast forward to 2024; by eliminating sugars, carb heavy and processed foods, this has been life-changing in so many ways. My weight, inflammation, joint pain and overall health has been positively transformed.

I sincerely hope by sharing my experiences it will help others too.

Peggy :)

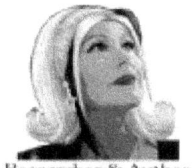

Researcher & Author
Peggy Annear

NoSugarNoGrain.Com

Do you have questions or comments?
Send me an email | peggyannear@nosugarnograin.com

Our Sugar Addiction Problem

The American Heart Association recommends that women should restrict their daily intake of added sugars to 25 grams (equivalent to approx 6 tsps), and for men, the limit is 37.5 grams (about 9 tsps). Surprisingly, studies indicate that in Western countries, we typically consume an average of 35 tsps of sugar daily.

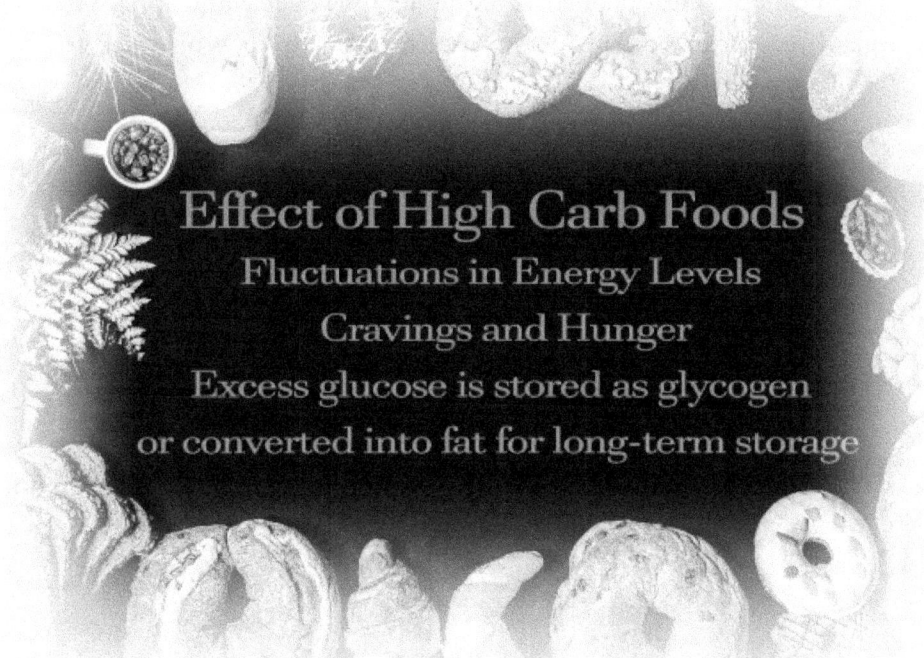

This excessive sugar consumption can be attributed to the pervasive **presence of hidden sugars in the majority of supermarket-bought foods**. It is much more complex than you adding 2 sugars to your coffee, or eating that sugar donut at breakfast time.

How this book will help you learn about insulin and HOW to eliminate hidden high- sugar, high-carbohydrate foods from your diet. These systematically bring on hunger pangs between meals. But when you conquer cravings, it puts you in control.

❖ Receive 7 days of low carb recipes with additional low GI ingredient options adding variety to suit your lifestyle.

❖ Understand which vegetables and fruits are best on a no sugar diet using the detailed list of Low- Sugar Vegetables and Low Sugar Fruits information.

❖ Discover how to read Nutrition labels on foods and identify harmful hidden sugars.

❖ Receive PDF Guides: Meal Planner, Shopping List Notes, and The printable meal planner & shopping organizer will help you to plan, record and create meals, inspiring you to keep on track to achieving your goals.

Our Focus

A favorite quote of mine is **"Give a man a fish, and you feed him for a day. Teach a man to fish, and you feed him for a lifetime"**. Once you have the knowledge of how to identify unhealthy sugary foods **you're essentially teaching yourself to fish, ensuring long-term well-being and nutritional awareness.**

Along with 7 days of healthy meals with total carb reduction, in this book you will discover the solution and focus on how to prevent insulin spikes, avoid hunger during meal times, and navigate sugar detox while decoding hidden sugars in food labels. You won't be hungry, simply learning to adjust what you eat and when.

Adopting a sensible approach to sugar management in our diet is crucial. People choose to follow a sugar-restricted diet for a range of reasons, such as weight loss, diabetes control, lowering cholesterol and blood pressure, and increasing energy levels. By integrating natural (unprocessed), nutritionally dense foods into our diet, we can reduce cravings and attain a satisfying feeling of fullness.

Carb intake will come from vegetables opposed to processed breads, grains and cereals.

To My Body & Heart

with Love.

How Does Blood Sugar Work?

A high-carbohydrate diet can have a significant impact on insulin spikes and blood sugar levels. Here's how it works:

❖ **1. Carbohydrate Consumption** - When you consume carbohydrates, they are broken down into glucose (sugar) in your digestive system. **Glucose is then absorbed into your bloodstream, leading to an increase in blood sugar levels.**

❖ Insulin Release - To regulate blood sugar levels, your body releases a hormone called insulin from the pancreas. Insulin's primary role is to perform the uptake of glucose into cells, where it can be used for energy or stored for later use. In a high-carb meal, your body releases more insulin, causing glucose spikes.

❖ Glycemic Index (GI) measures how quickly a carb-containing food raises blood sugar levels: Low GI (55 or less) foods cause a slow, gradual rise in blood sugar, promoting stable energy.

High GI (70 or more) foods **lead to a rapid, significant increase in blood sugar, often causing energy spikes and crashes.** Hence low GI foods and beverages assist to stabilize blood sugar, promoting sustained energy, and reduces the risk of chronic diseases.

❖ Insulin Spikes - High-carb meals can cause a rapid and substantial increase in blood sugar levels, which, in turn, leads to a corresponding spike in insulin release. This is known as an "insulin spike." The goal of this spike is to move excess glucose out of the bloodstream and into cells.

❖ Blood Sugar Regulation - As insulin works to bring blood sugar levels back to normal, the excess glucose is either stored in the liver and muscles as glycogen or converted into fat for long-term storage.

This process helps prevent blood sugar from reaching dangerous levels, but it can lead to fluctuations in energy levels and hunger.

Here are the key effects of a high-carb diet on insulin and blood sugar levels:

❖ Blood Sugar Peaks and Crashes - High-carb meals can cause blood sugar to rise quickly, leading to an energy boost (a "sugar high"). However, this is often followed by **a crash in blood sugar levels, which can result in fatigue, cravings for more carbohydrates, and irritability.**

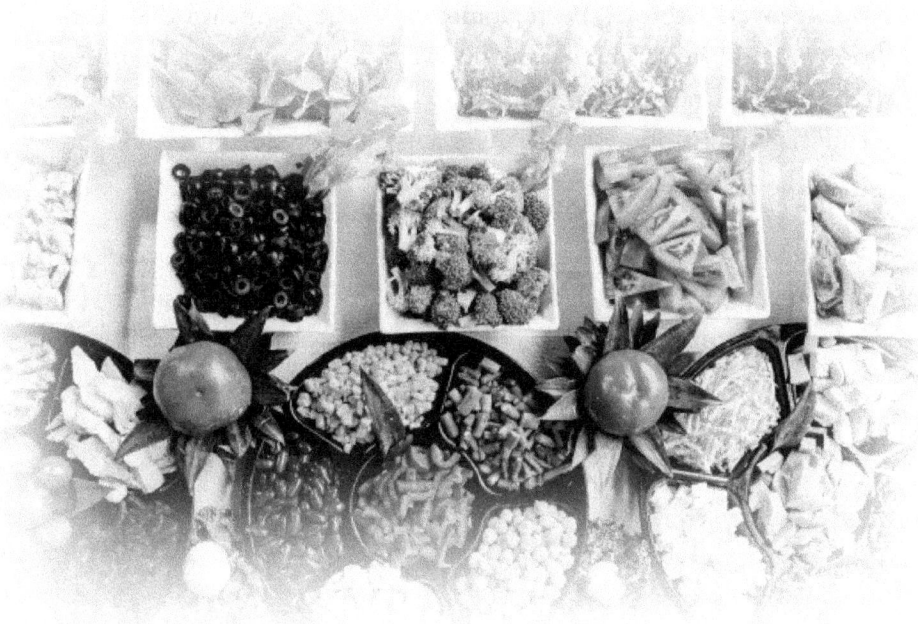

❖ **Increased Insulin Resistance** - Consistently consuming a diet high in carbohydrates, especially refined and simple sugars, can lead to increased insulin resistance. This means that your cells become less responsive to insulin's signals, and your pancreas may have to produce even more insulin to keep blood sugar levels in check.

❖ **Weight Gain - Excess glucose that is not used for immediate energy or stored as glycogen can be converted into fat and stored in adipose tissue**. Over time, a high-carb diet, especially one that exceeds your energy expenditure, can contribute to weight gain.

❖ Risk of Type 2 Diabetes - **Prolonged exposure to high levels of blood sugar and insulin spikes can increase the risk of developing type 2 diabetes.** In this condition, the body's ability to regulate blood sugar effectively is compromised.

- ❖ **Improved Athletic Performance** - While high-carb diets can lead to blood sugar fluctuations in everyday life, athletes often use carb-loading strategies to enhance performance, as the body's stores of glycogen can be a significant energy source during prolonged physical activity.

As you can see the effects of a high-carb diet can vary among each of us and our energy output, and factors such as the type of carbohydrates consumed (simple vs. complex), portion sizes, and overall dietary balance play a crucial role.

Are Carbs and Sugars Equal?

While all sugars are carbohydrates, not all carbohydrates are sugars.

Carbohydrates encompass a broader category of compounds, including both simple sugars and complex carbohydrates like starch and fiber.

Removing added sugars from our diet in the form of excess carbs is the quickest way to lose weight and increase energy levels. Out of balance blood sugar levels can cause depression which encourages the body to store sugar as fat instead of using it for energy. The sugar detox plan aims to remove sugars and simple carbohydrates from your diet. **Your skin, dental health and mental focus will benefit too!** Vegetables and salads are rich in complex carbs and fibre. We will be detoxing or cleansing important organs of the body such as the liver, kidneys and colon of accumulated wastes and toxins.

The cravings for carb dense foods and sugar will start subsiding after about 5 - 7 days for most people. The good news is the longer you stay off sugar, the easier it gets. The detox will correct or stabilize your sugar levels, then you can add small amounts of fruits and healthy wholegrain breads back into your diet if you wish.

It's not possible to see added sugars in teaspoons on packaging during manufacturing, but the Nutrition Facts label on a food can help us to identify added sugars. Look for common sweeteners such as sucrose/sugar, corn syrup, glucose and dextrose.

Consumption of added sugars, including sucrose, can have negative health effects. Here are some more considerations why balanced low carb is better:

*Dental Health - Sucrose can promote tooth decay and cavities when consumed in sugary snacks and beverages. Bacteria in the mouth feed on sugars and produce acids that can erode tooth enamel.

*Blood Sugar - Sucrose can cause a rapid spike in blood sugar levels when consumed in large quantities, especially when not paired with fiber or other nutrients and fats. This can lead to insulin resistance and, over time, increase the risk of type 2 diabetes.

*Cardiovascular Health - Excessive sugar intake, including sucrose, has been linked to increased risk of heart disease and high blood pressure.

*Fatty Liver Disease - High sugar consumption, especially from fructose (which is one component of sucrose), has been associated with non-alcoholic fatty liver disease.

*Sugar Addiction - It is widely accepted amongst medical professionals that sugar can be addictive, leading to cravings and overconsumption. (This is also true for salt).

Many of us have become trapped in the modern food cycle of eating sugary foods without a second thought. We can feel depressed and don't know how to get off the "sugar ride". The good news is that quitting sugar and detoxifying the body is quite a fast process. The physical dependence on carbs can be eliminated in only five to seven days by avoiding sugar and sugary foods altogether. During these five to seven days you'll learn how to beat cravings.

There is **NO NEED to feel hungry**, simply adjust food choices and the time you eat.

You will learn tips on how to quit sugar and beat the cravings. **Once you have knowledge on how to identify unhealthy sugary foods** you can easily plan your journey ahead on a sugar-free lifestyle that will have your body feeling amazingly good.

What is a Detox Diet?

Detox diets generally refer to the restriction or elimination of processed foods, sugar, and other potentially harmful substances such as unhealthy fats, artificial food preservatives, flavorings and additives etc. This commonly leads to reduced inflammation in the body, improved heart & brain health, weight loss and improved gut health. **We'll be eating "real foods"** that stop cravings. For maintaining long term good health we are primarily focusing on carb and sugar detox, while paying special attention to these other important factors as well.

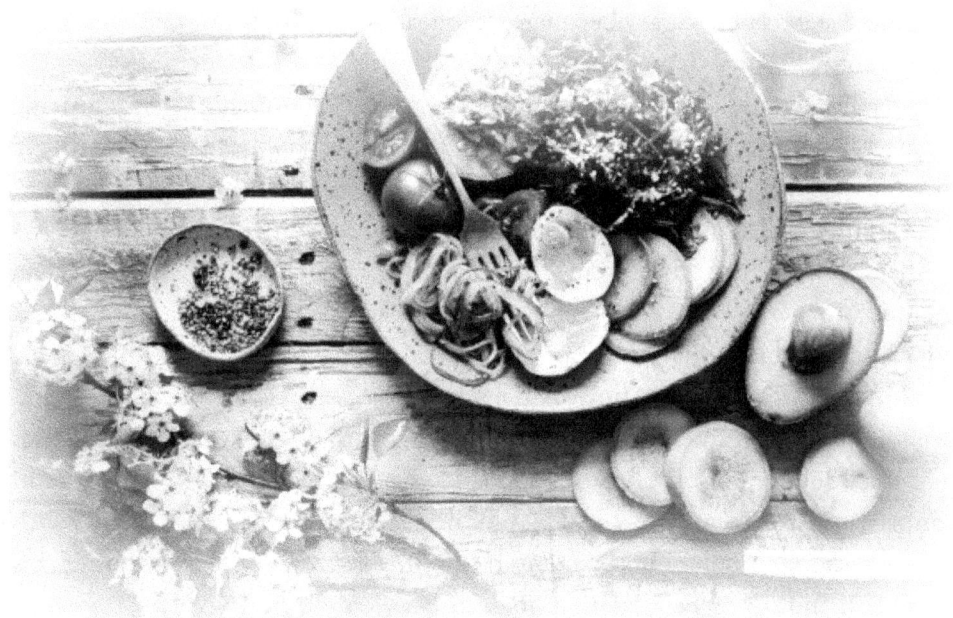

How Quitting Sugar Will Change Your Life

Weight Management - Some people use detox diets to "kick-start" a longer term strategy for weight loss. High sugar diets are often linked to weight gain and obesity. Excess body fat can produce inflammatory substances, contributing to chronic inflammation. By quitting sugar or reducing sugar intake, you can better manage your weight and decrease the inflammation associated with obesity.

Improved Digestion - Proponents who have experienced detox diets (like me) argue that they can help improve digestive health by giving the digestive system a break, promoting the
consumption of high-quality and fiber foods that help improve gut health.

Reduced Inflammation - Added sugars, especially in the form of sucrose (table sugar) and high-fructose corn syrup, have been associated with an increase in inflammatory markers in the body. Excessive sugar consumption can lead to chronic, low-grade inflammation, which is believed to be a contributing factor in the development and progression of various inflammatory diseases, including conditions like arthritis, heart disease, and inflammatory bowel disease.

Improved Insulin Sensitivity - High sugar intake, especially in the form of refined sugars and sugary beverages, can lead to insulin resistance, which is a risk factor for type 2 diabetes.

Insulin resistance is associated with chronic inflammation. By reducing sugar consumption, you can improve insulin sensitivity, potentially reducing inflammation.

Balanced Gut Microbiota - High sugar diets can negatively affect the composition of the gut microbiota. Dysbiosis in the gut can trigger an inflammatory response. Reducing sugar intake may help balance the gut microbiota and reduce inflammation.

Lowered Risk of Metabolic Syndrome - Excessive sugar consumption has been linked to an increased risk of metabolic syndrome, a cluster of conditions that include high blood pressure, high blood sugar, excess abdominal fat, and abnormal cholesterol levels. Metabolic syndrome is associated with inflammation, so reducing sugar intake can lower the risk of developing this condition and the associated inflammation.

Reduced Oxidative Stress - Sugar consumption, particularly in high amounts, can lead to oxidative stress in the body. Oxidative stress is linked to inflammation and various chronic diseases. Cutting back on sugar can help reduce oxidative stress.

Improved Immune Function - High sugar intake can suppress the immune system's function, making the body more susceptible to infections and inflammatory conditions. Reducing sugar consumption can help support a healthier immune system.

The human body has its own built-in mechanisms for detoxification, primarily involving the liver, kidneys, and other organs. Extreme long term radical detox diets can be harmful, leading to nutritional deficiencies, muscle loss, and a slowed metabolism.

Instead, we are working towards a long term healthier solution that will help regulate your appetite and prevent feelings of hunger shortly after eating. Stabilizing your insulin levels helps to beat hunger cravings between meals.

When you reduce sugars and carbs, your body enters a state of ketosis, where it shifts from using glucose as its primary fuel to burning stored fat for energy. This metabolic transition produces ketones, which serve as an alternative fuel source for the brain and other tissues. Reducing sugars and going into ketosis can have positive effects on the body for many people, as it promotes fat burning and may contribute to weight loss. Additionally, it can help stabilize blood sugar levels and improve insulin sensitivity, potentially benefiting those with conditions like type 2 diabetes.

We all have a different body size, calories expended, and some with special health conditions. Before embarking on any radical diet or making significant changes to your eating habits, it's a good idea to consult with a healthcare professional or your dietitian. They can help you make informed decisions about your dietary choices and ensure that any changes you make align with your overall health goals.

In replacement of an extreme crazy low calorie detox diet, we'll be focusing on a balanced and sustainable approach to clean eating and nutrition. This is recommended for long- term health and general well-being.

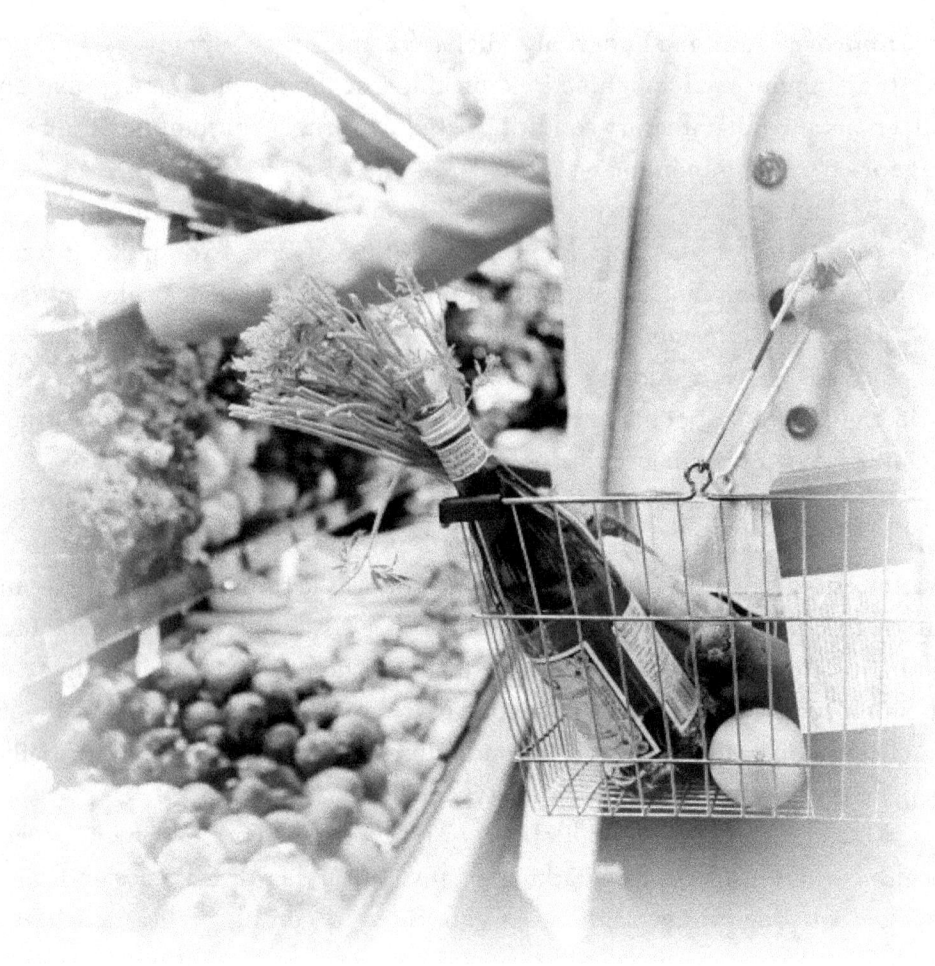

In doing so, **you will be in control and have the power and understanding to make informed decisions, enabling you to reach your goals.**

It is a learning process; hang in there, and you will be on a journey of learning about the many hidden tricks that processed foods contain.

How Snacking Effects Insulin

Constant and excessive spikes in insulin due to frequent snacking on high sugar or high carb foods can lead to insulin resistance over time. Insulin resistance can increase the risk of type 2 diabetes and other health issues.

Rapid insulin spikes can lead to a quick drop in blood sugar, *which can trigger feelings of hunger shortly after eating.* This can make it challenging to manage calorie intake and body weight. This is why snacking of all carb dense foods are eradicated during detox and suggested post detox too. For this reason low sugar fruits may be added with a meal but only in strict moderation after detox.

Chronic **high insulin levels are associated with increased inflammation**, which can contribute to various health problems, including cardiovascular disease and arthritis.

To summarize, while insulin spikes are a normal part of the body's response to food, frequent and excessive spikes, particularly from high-sugar or high-carb foods, can have negative consequences. It's recommended to consume balanced meals with a mix of carbohydrates (as mostly vegetables and salads), proteins, and healthy fats to help maintain stable blood sugar levels and prevent excessive insulin spikes. Moreover, it's essential to consider your activity level such as heavy exercise, dietary needs and the impact of insulin between meals.

This is why including **a small amount of complex carbs protein and healthy fats is crucial in controlling insulin levels.** Feelings of hunger won't be triggered after eating.

Your metabolism will run smoothly and you'll have more energy!

Of course, if you have specific concerns about your insulin levels or blood sugar management always speak with your Doctor or Holistic Specialist or Nutritionist.

How Artificial Sweeteners Differ

Artificial sweeteners may not be a long term solution to removing table and cooking sugar. However as you retrain your taste buds they are useful and help to reduce your dependence. Note; using large amounts of artificial sweeteners may lead to adverse health side effects. Over time you will start finding that artificial sweeteners taste unpalatable and way too sweet! Stevia and Agave seem to be popular natural plant based sweeteners around right now, however Agave is very high in fructose. Stevia is my personal choice in moderation.

Beware of Chemical Sweeteners

These "chemical" sweeteners are often used to reduce the calorie content of products and cater to consumers looking for sugar-free or low-calorie options. Some examples of artificial sweeteners commonly found in supermarket foods include:

***Aspartame** - Found in many sugar-free or "diet" products, including diet sodas, sugar-free gum, and sugar-free desserts.

***Sucralose** - Often used in sugar-free and "light" products like diet drinks, sugar-free syrups, and some baked goods.

***Saccharin** - Used in sugar-free sweeteners, diet sodas, and some tabletop sweeteners.

***Acesulfame Potassium (Ace-K)** - Found in a variety of sugar-free and "diet" products, including beverages, sugar-free gum, and sugar-free desserts.

***Neotame** - A newer artificial sweetener used in some low- calorie and sugar-free products.

***Cyclamate** - Though banned in some countries due to safety concerns, it is still used in certain foods and beverages in others.

***Advantame** - A high-intensity artificial sweetener, similar to aspartame, used in some sugar-free products.

***Allulose** - Although not an artificial sweetener, allulose is a low- calorie sugar substitute that occurs naturally in small amounts in
some foods. It is used in some sugar-free and low-calorie products.

***Sorbitol** - Sorbitol is another sugar alcohol used in various sugar-free or reduced-sugar products, including sugar-free candies and chewing gum.

Although deemed safe, unfortunately has been known to upset digestion especially in IBS sufferers. (Irritable Bowel Syndrome) Some common sense has to come into play with sweeteners.

Moderation is key. However you won't be craving sugar like you did before detox, so you will only want limited sweetness as days progress.

Opting for small portions of Stevia extract, monk fruit, Xylitol, or natural honey, or maple syrup in controlled moderation (the later two only post detox!) is a wiser choice rather than reverting back to consuming sugar. Likewise with processed 'sugar-free' supermarket products loaded with artificial sweeteners and additives, which are detrimental to health.

At the time of writing, the following sweetener powders and extracts are popular and **deemed safe**. (More on this in the next section)

***Stevia** - A natural safe sweetener derived from the leaves of the stevia plant, it is often used as a sugar substitute in various foods and beverages.

***Monk Fruit** - A newer natural sweetener derived from mogroside, which is the sweetest part of the fruit.

***Xylitol: Xylitol** - A natural sweetener from sugar alcohol from fruits. It has a similar sweetness to table sugar but with fewer calories.

GI Spikes and Fructose

The Glycemic Index is known as GI. **GI ranks carbohydrate-containing foods based on how quickly they raise blood sugar.**

It's a scale from 0 to 100; higher values mean a rapid blood sugar increase.

High-GI foods (e.g. white bread & sweets) cause quick spikes, while low-GI foods (e.g. whole grains) lead to gradual increases which is good for metabolic balance.

*GI mainly applies to carb-containing foods.

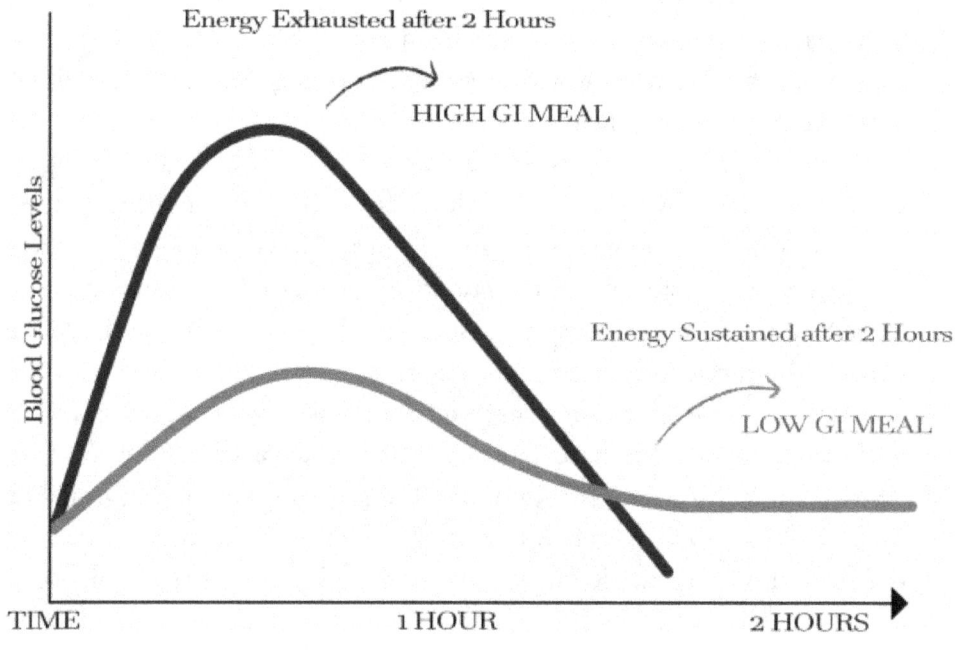

Fructose is a simple sugar found in fruits, some veggies, table sugar (sucrose), and high-fructose corn syrup (HFCS). When consumed, the liver metabolizes fructose, which has a low glycemic response. **Excessive fructose, especially from added sugars, can lead to health issues like obesity and fatty liver.**

The link between GI and Fructose

Foods with fructose can have a low GI due to the slower release of fructose into the bloodstream.

*Fruits have a low to moderate GI because of their fiber content, which slows fructose absorption.

*__GI is influenced by factors like fiber and fat content.__ A fruit salad with more fiber may have a lower GI than pure fruit juice, despite both containing fructose.

Consider a food's complete nutritional profile and volume before consuming - including carbs, fiber, and fat, to assess its blood sugar impact and overall health.

Fructose typically has a lower glycemic response than glucose, but the GI of foods can vary due to factors beyond fructose content. It's important to consider both GI and fructose content when making dietary choices, especially for blood sugar management.

Don't forget too, certain recipes can be adapted by reducing sugar and substituting sugar with Stevia or Monk fruit. In their pure forms they are almost calorie-free and have no grams of sugar. However, it's essential to **read product labels, especially for blended or processed versions of any food including these sweeteners,** to ensure you are getting the desired level of sweetness without added calories or sugars.

After detox, in place of sugar you may try honey, maple syrup (or dates) as these are natural, but have approx 5-7 gms of sugar in glucose and fructose per tsp. This consolidates that home cooked is usually better than store bought because you know what goes into each recipe! Your homemade recipes will be free of all those nasty added sugars, chemical additives and preservatives.

Fresh Fruit vs Dried Fruit Example - The sugar content in dried prunes are much higher than that in fresh plums due to the removal of water during the drying process. Dried prunes are essentially dehydrated plums, which concentrates the sugars.

Fresh Plum - A medium-sized fresh plum (about 2.5 inches in diameter) typically contains Approx. 8-10 grams of sugar.

Dried Prune - One dried prune, on the other hand, contains around 2-3 grams of sugar. However, because they've lost their water content during the drying process, dried prunes are much smaller and more calorie-dense than fresh plums.

While the sugar content is lower per prune, it's important to be mindful of volume and portion sizes when consuming dried fruits, as **it's easy to eat a larger quantity compared to fresh fruits**, which can result in a significant sugar intake and calories.

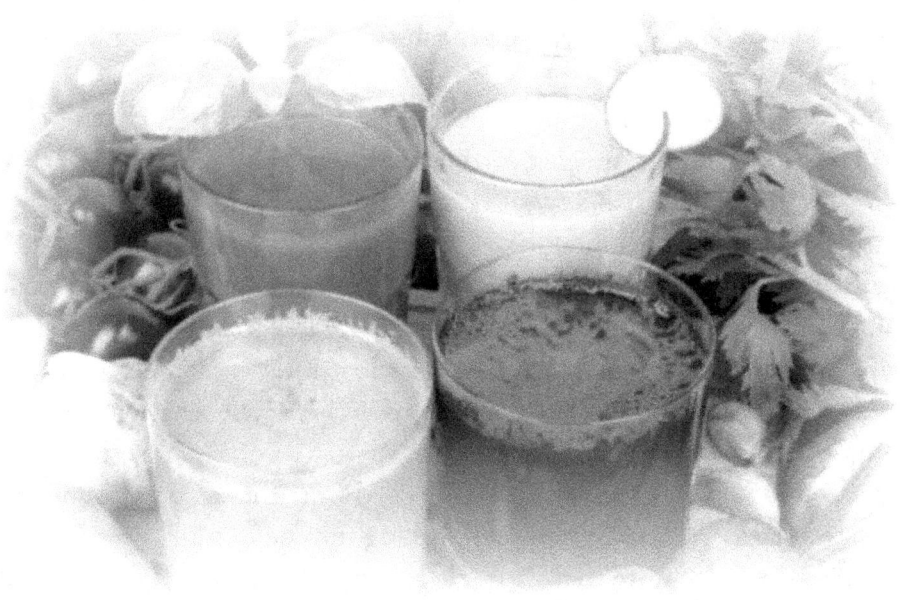

To recap the sweetener options

Safe natural sweeteners are sweetening agents derived from natural sources that are considered safe for consumption.

Some commonly used safe natural sweeteners include:

Stevia - Stevia is a sweet herb native to South America. It is known for its intense sweetness without calories. Steviol glycosides, the compounds responsible for the sweetness, are extracted from the leaves and used as a sweetener. (This is my favourite, I only use about 1/10th tsp in black tea)

Monk Fruit - Monk fruit extract, also known as luo han guo, is derived from a fruit native to Southeast Asia. It is extremely sweet and has no calories. Monk fruit extract contains natural antioxidants and is considered safe for most people.

Erythritol - Erythritol is a sugar alcohol that occurs naturally in some fruits and fermented foods. It has a sweet taste with very few calories and does not significantly impact blood sugar levels.

Xylitol - Xylitol is another sugar alcohol found in small amounts in some fruits and vegetables. It has a similar sweetness to table sugar but with fewer calories. Xylitol is often used as a sugar substitute and has been shown to have dental health benefits.

Yacon Syrup - Yacon syrup is extracted from the roots of the yacon plant, which is native to South America. It contains fructooligosaccharides, which are a type of soluble fiber with a sweet taste. Yacon syrup is lower in calories and has a minimal impact on blood sugar levels.

Maple Syrup/Honey (in moderation) - While maple syrup and honey are natural sweeteners, they should be consumed only in moderation, but not during detox. Both contain high amounts of natural sugars as glucose and fructose. They do provide calories, but they also contain beneficial compounds like antioxidants and minerals.

Coconut Sugar - Coconut sugar is derived from the sap of coconut palm trees. It is used as a natural sweetener in baking and cooking.

It's important to **note that while these natural sweeteners are generally considered safe for most people, individual tolerance and dietary needs may vary**. Additionally, some natural sweeteners may have a distinct taste or aftertaste that may not be preferred by everyone. Always consult with your

Doctor or nutritionist if you have specific dietary concerns or specific health conditions.

Soluble Fiber vs Insoluble Fiber

Research has explored the effects of different types of dietary fiber on sugar absorption, particularly carbohydrate metabolism and blood sugar levels. Soluble fiber has been shown to have certain benefits.

Soluble fiber, found in foods like chia, oats, legumes, and some fruits, forms a gel-like substance when mixed with water. This gel can slow down the digestion and absorption of carbohydrates, which may help regulate blood sugar levels. It can also affect the absorption of sugars, such as glucose, in the digestive tract. In regard to oats, it is not recommended on a low carb diet, however it would be considered a better option compared to bread.

Insoluble fiber, found in foods like whole grains and vegetables, does not dissolve in water and generally passes through the digestive system relatively intact. While it doesn't directly impact sugar absorption, insoluble fiber is valuable for digestive health and can contribute to a feeling of fullness, potentially helping with weight management.

Soluble fiber supports digestive health by forming a gel-like substance that slows down digestion, fostering a sense of fullness and potentially assisting in weight management. (Chia seeds featured in our recipes here) Additionally, it plays a role in blood sugar regulation by slowing down the absorption of sugars from the digestive tract. In contrast, insoluble fiber contributes to digestive health by adding bulk to the stool, preventing constipation, and promoting regular bowel movements. It also aids in weight management by enhancing the feeling of fullness.

Therefore soluble fiber, due to its ability to form a gel-like substance helps the slowing down of absorption and digestion so is related to the concept of a lower Glycemic Index (GI). This is due to how quickly a carbohydrate containing food raises blood glucose levels. **Foods with a low GI are digested and absorbed more slowly, leading to a slower and more gradual increase in blood sugar levels.**

Contributing to a lower glycemic response is beneficial, especially for people wanting to manage their blood sugar levels and those aiming for sustained energy levels.

How Controlling Insulin Levels Boosts Fat Loss

Insulin is a hormone produced by the pancreas that plays a crucial role in regulating blood sugar (glucose) levels. **When we eat carbohydrates, especially those with a high glycemic index, they are broken down into glucose, causing an increase in blood sugar levels.** In response to this rise in blood sugar, the pancreas releases insulin to help cells absorb and use the glucose for energy or store it for future use.

Insulin has several functions, one of which is to promote the storage of excess glucose as glycogen in the liver and muscles. **However, if these storage sites are already full, the excess glucose is converted into fat** and stored in adipose tissue. This process is part of the body's natural energy storage mechanism.

Now, when insulin levels are frequently elevated due to a diet high in refined carbohydrates and sugars, it can lead to a state of insulin resistance. In insulin resistance, cells become less responsive to the effects of insulin, and the pancreas produces even more insulin to compensate. This increased insulin production is associated with various metabolic issues, including an increased tendency to store fat and a reduced ability to burn stored fat for energy.

Here's why insulin spikes can be problematic for weight loss:

Fat Storage - Elevated insulin levels promote the storage of excess glucose as fat, contributing to weight gain.

Reduced Fat Burning - Insulin inhibits the breakdown of stored fat for energy. When insulin levels are high, the body is less efficient at using fat as a fuel source.

Increased Hunger - Insulin spikes can lead to fluctuations in blood sugar levels, which may result in increased hunger and cravings, making it more challenging to stick to a calorie-controlled diet.

Energy Imbalance - Constant insulin spikes can contribute to an imbalance between energy intake and expenditure, favoring fat storage.

This is why not overeating combined with a no sugar low carb diet will contribute in a major way to your weight loss efforts as well as better health generally. You don't need to be hungry, rather eat the right foods at the right time.

Green juices can help support weight loss through their low-calorie content, nutrient density, hydration contribution, **fiber presence (helping reduce carbs to net carbs)**, potential for natural detoxification, and reduced processed sugar intake.

Eat as many leafy greens, celery and other low carb vegetables as you wish as these do not spike insulin and make you hungry. All are extremely low (around 1-3 grams) in carbohydrates and sugars.

The Exercise Myth; You've Been Lied to...Here's the Truth

Here is an example for demonstration purposes. We see it everywhere...exercise to lose X amount of weight, ads showing workout exercise machines and sculpted bodies. However what these ads fail to tell you is that exercise is only a small and often misunderstood part of the weight loss equation. Diet matters...a lot.

The Calorie Equation

Calorie Surplus: If your calorie intake exceeds the calories you burn through metabolism and activity, you are in a caloric surplus. This can lead to weight gain as the excess calories are stored as fat.

Caloric Deficit. If your calorie expenditure exceeds your intake, you are in a caloric deficit. This situation can result in weight loss, as your body taps into stored energy (fat) to meet its energy needs.

Caloric Maintenance. When calorie intake equals expenditure, your weight remains relatively stable. This is referred to as caloric maintenance.

The Weight Management Equation

➤ **Weight Loss:** Caloric deficit (calories burned > calories consumed)

➤ **Weight Maintenance:** Caloric balance (calories burned = calories consumed)

➤ **Weight Gain:** Caloric surplus (calories consumed > calories burned)

Consider the following...

Quality of Your Calorie Intake. While the quantity of calories is essential, the quality of the calories (nutrient density) also matters for overall health.

Individual Variation: The ideal balance between calorie intake and exercise can vary based on factors such as metabolism, age, gender, and activity level.

Calorie Intake and Requirements. The average calorie intake for women aged 25-55 can vary based on factors such as activity level, metabolism, height, weight, and overall health. However, there are general guidelines provided by health authorities.

The Dietary Guidelines for Americans suggest a daily calorie intake range based on age, sex, and physical activity level. They recommend;

Women with little to no exercise About 1,800 to 2,000 calories per day.

Moderately Active Women (engaging in physical activity equivalent to walking 1.5 to 3 (4.8km) miles at a pace of 3 to 4 miles per hour) About 2,000 to 2,200 calories per day.

Active Women (engaging in physical activity equivalent to walking to 2,400 calories per day.

That is a lot of walking to burn calories! These are general guidelines, and individual calorie intake varies. It's essential to consider factors such as muscle mass, metabolism, and specific health goals.

Here are approximate values for the number of calories burned per hour for different activities based on a person weighing around 155-160 pounds (70-73 kg):

-**Walking** (3.5 mph): About 314 calories per hour.

more than 3 miles (4.8km) per day at the same pace): About 2,200

-**Running** (5 mph): About 590 calories per hour.

-**Cycling** (12-14 mph): About 472 calories per hour.

-**Swimming** (moderate intensity): About 413 calories per hour.

-**Aerobic Exercise** (general): About 413 calories per hour.

-**Strength Training** About 236 calories per hour.

Exercise and fitness play a big part in our overall physical fitness and mental health.

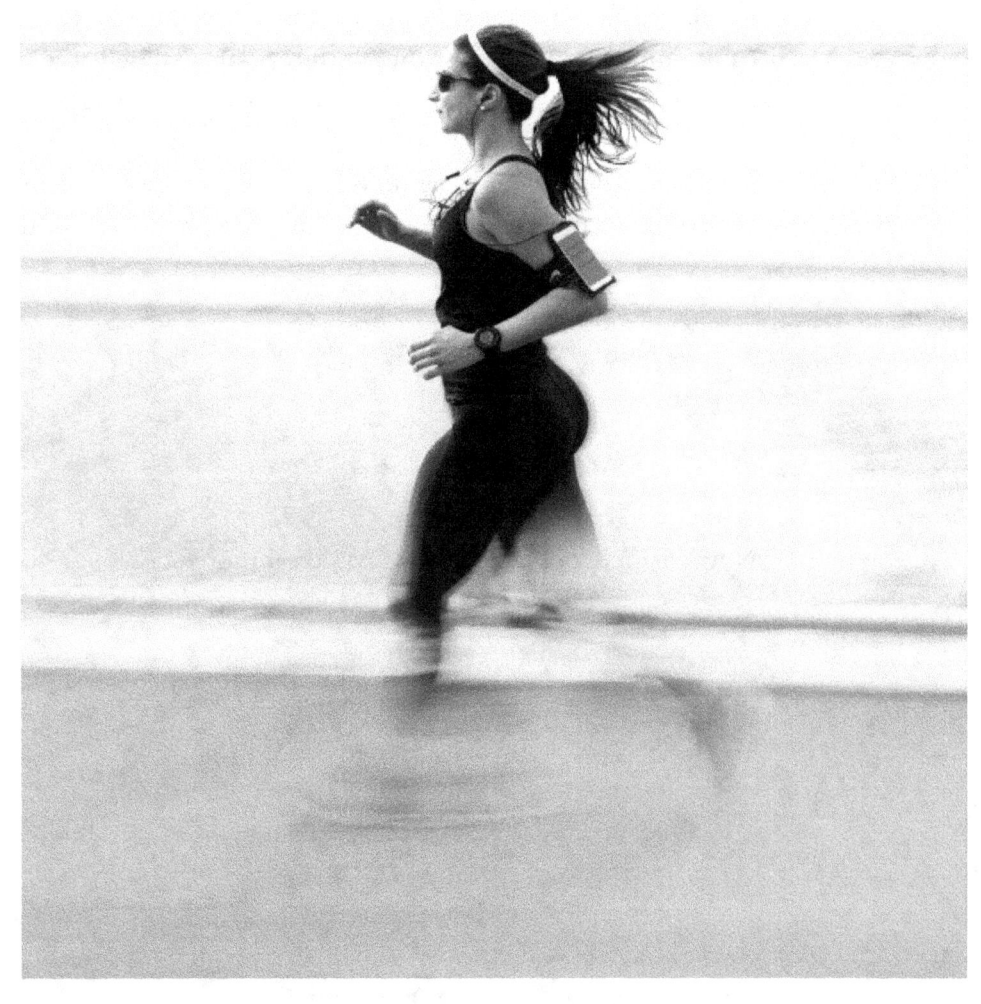

Exercise releases endorphins and dopamine, promoting a sense of well-being and happiness. In addition to this, exercise is beneficial for toning your body as you lose body fat.

Incorporating strength training into a weight loss program not only burns calories during the workout but also boosts your metabolism, preserves muscle mass, and promotes a better body composition by reducing fat while increasing lean muscle tissue.

In summary, both diet and exercise are important for weight loss and maintaining overall health, **however diet plays a more crucial role.** Research suggests that combining a caloric deficit diet with regular exercise is the most effective approach for weight loss, weight maintenance, and overall health benefits like improved cardiovascular fitness, glycemic control, and mental well-being. While diet is the biggest driver of weight loss, exercise complements dietary changes to optimize weight management and promote holistic health.

NOTES

Nutrient-rich low sugar foods I could eat more of ...

Preparing for the 7 Day Elimination Plan

A 7-day carb food detox plan is a short-term dietary regimen designed to help cleanse the body, promote healthier eating habits, improve energy and potentially jumpstart weight loss. Consuming too many carbohydrates makes energy levels erratic, can quickly spike blood sugar levels which may cause problems over time leading to diabetes and/or high blood pressure.

Monitoring and maintaining carbohydrate intake is key to blood sugar control. Closely scrutinizing processed packaged and bottled foods from the supermarket during detox and afterwards is recommended.

Remove foods with high GI sugary carbohydrates

*These include sugary beverages, processed foods, breads and dairy, desserts, dried fruits, sweets, candy, honey, syrups and high sugar fruits.

*Foods high in starchy carbohydrates include starchy vegetables, flour based foods including cereals, peas and beans to a lesser extent, and whole grains such as white rice, barley, oats and quinoa.

In preparation for low carb no sugar food shopping, I've created this quick checklist reminder which I hope you find useful:

Download available[1] at my website NoSugarNoGrain.Com

---

1. https://nosugarnograin.com/low-carb-sugar-list-grocery-checklist-planner/

LOW SUGAR GROCERY CHECKLIST

Basics For A No Sugar Diet

- [ ] **LOW SUGAR VEGETABLES**
- [ ] **WHOLE FOODS & EGGS**
- [ ] **QUALITY MEATS | ORGANIC**
- [ ] **LOW SUGAR SAUCES & OILS**
- [ ] **UNPROCESSED FOODS**
- [ ] **LEAFY GREENS**
- [ ] **FULL FAT DAIRY**
- [ ] **UNSWEETENED NUT MILKS**
- [ ] **LOW SUGAR FRUITS**
- [ ] **HEALTHY NUTS & SEEDS**

NO JUNK FOODS

NOSUGARNOGRAIN.COM

How to Read Food Labels for Weight Loss

Locate the "Nutritional Information" on the food packaging. **Look for "Total Carbohydrates" and "Sugars"** as both these will be indicated there. (Keep in mind that trans fats are unhealthy) Remember Fructose and Corn Syrup are among the worst offenders! **Your goal is to aim for foods lower than 5g if possible. Analyze the sugar content per 100g, as serving sizes can vary between products.**

Nutrient	Per Serv	Per 100g
Calories (kcal)	130.85	307.7
Calories from Fat (kcal)	28.66	67.39
Fat (g)	3.22	7.58
Saturated Fat (g)	0.61	1.44
Trans Fatty Acid (g)	0.01	0.01
Cholesterol (mg)	0	0
Carbohydrates (g)	21.8	51.27
Dietary Fiber (g)	1.97	4.63
Total Sugars (g)	0.74	1.74
Protein (g)	3.44	8.09
Mono Fat (g)	0.53	1.25

The goal for diabetics, whether or not they use insulin, is to keep their blood sugar as steady as possible and to maximize their intake of nutritious carbs and minimize consumption of less nutritious foods. A starting place for diabetics is to have roughly 45 to 60g of carbs per meal and 15 to 30g for snacks. Consult your doctor.

What is an Acceptable Amount of Sugar?

- ❖ **High – over 22g of total sugars per 100g**
- ❖ **Low – 5g of total sugars or less per 100g**

*If the amount of sugars per 100g is between these figures, then levels of sugar match accordingly.

*The sugar amount in the nutrition label is the **total amount of sugars in the food**. It includes added sugars and sugars from ingredients such as fruits and milk.

Is Fiber Relevant to Blood Sugar Levels?
Yes! The presence of **dietary fiber in a food item can reduce the effective carbohydrate content because fiber is not digested and absorbed** in the same way as other carbohydrates. Since fiber is not metabolized into glucose, **it has a minimal impact on blood sugar levels.** The calculation is as follows:

Net Carbs = Total Carbs − Fiber

You may apply this equation to all recipes. In this example image Total Carbs are 51.27 gm, dietary fiber is 4.63 gm. So 51.27 minus 4.6 = 46.67. **Therefore the Net Carbs are 46.67**

What is an Acceptable Amount of Carbohydrates?

The Dietary Guidelines for Americans recommend that carbohydrates make up about 45-65% of total daily calories.

However a common range for carbohydrate intake on a low-carb diet is typically between 20% and 50% of total daily calories. A low-carb detox diet with a carb target of < 50 grams of carbohydrates per day will be a viable approach for some, particularly when aiming for weight loss or blood sugar control. For others <80gm carbs per day would be more suitable depending on your energy output.

The Math: How to Calculate Percentage of Calories From Carbohydrates

We need to find out how many grams of carbohydrates you have in a day. For example, one sweet potato contains 26 grams of carbs, says the USDA. Do this by breaking down every recipe or food you eat. Check labels. Once you have the number of grams of carbs you took in, you can multiply it by 4 as there are 4 calories in every gram of carbs. If you had 200 grams of carbohydrates in a day, that would equate to 800 of your daily calories from carbohydrates. You can then calculate the percentage of calories that came from carbs. Take the number of calories that came from carbohydrates and divide it by the total amount of calories you had in a day. Then multiply that number by 100 to get the percentage.

As described by The National Library of Medicine, carbohydrates are sugar molecules. The body breaks down carbs as the main source of energy for cells, tissues and organs. Micronutrients (required in smaller amounts) are essential minerals required in small amounts for vital physiological functions. Examples include iron, zinc, and calcium, all playing crucial roles in metabolism, immune function, and bone health.

We will be primarily getting these through vegetables, leafy greens, nuts and seeds. Macronutrients (required in larger amounts) are the proteins, fats and carbs your body needs the most in order to function because our body can't make enough on its own. For proper nutrition it's crucial we get them from our diet.

Food Choices

1. To focus on carbohydrate restriction we'll be eliminating high-carb foods, including sugars, grains, starchy veggies, along with most fruits.

2. To compensate for reduced carbs we'll replace them with an increase of healthy fat intake from avocados, nuts, seeds, olive oil, and fatty fish.

3. Proteins will be included in moderation from meat, poultry, fish, eggs and low carb dairy.

When comparing white and whole-wheat bread, it's worth noting they can have similar carbohydrate content, but whole-wheat bread is often a better choice due to its complex carbs, lower glycemic index (GI). Keep in mind that the exact carbohydrate content can vary between brands and types of bread, so always refer to the nutrition label for precise information.

Some food labels don't display sugar per 100g. Always analyze the sugars and total carbs PLUS observe if it's only per Serving Size because that equates to a lot more of that ingredient.

Check the Total Carbohydrates in Foods. Sugars are a simple form of carbohydrates, which are one of the three main macronutrients (along with proteins and fats). Therefore, monitoring both sugar and overall carbohydrate intake is important.

Pumpkin (7gm carb per 100gm) is a better option than sweet and white potato (approx 18gm carbs per 100gm).

Quinoa may have only 0.9g of sugar per 100g, but has 64g of total carbs! It is also however high in fibre, so this is where a balanced diet full of a variety of natural foods is your best option for health and weight loss. Moderation is the key when eating high carb or high sugar foods. In saying that, all "junk" foods need to be removed altogether as they have virtually no nutritional value whatsoever!

I spotted this "health bar" package at the supermarket. It had a surprisingly high sugar content of 25g, and this measurement wasn't even based on 100g but on the serving size, which is just one bar! This contradicts the idea of a healthy choice and appears to be a tactic to make it seem like it contains less sugar. Additionally, it had 33g of total carbohydrates! On food labels, "sugars" refer to both naturally occurring sugars (e.g. those found in fruits and dairy) and added sugars (e.g. sucrose, high fructose corn syrup). So the question to ask is what natural food would be a contributor to these sugars, as they often come with other beneficial nutrients like fiber and vitamins. Eg you would think it only reasonable to have some natural sugars in say a can of whole plums, but not so much for a "health" bar.

Serving Size 1 Bar (85g)	
Servings Per Container 4	

Amount Per Serving	
Calories 170	Calories from Fat 50

	% Daily Value *
Total Fat 6g	9%
Saturated Fat 4g	19%
Trans Fat 0g	
Polyunsaturated Fat 0.5g	
Monounsaturated Fat 1g	
Cholesterol 13mg	4%
Sodium 83mg	3%
Total Carbohydrate 33g	11%
Dietary Fiber 4g	16%
Sugar 25g	
Protein 3g	

| Vitamin A 110% | • | Vitamin C 2% |
| Calcium 10% | • | Iron 3% |

Foods to Eat for Energy & Success

The goal is eliminating all sugary, carb-heavy foods during the 7-day sugar detox phase. You can prepare meat, poultry, or seafood and serve them with a salad or vegetables every day. Remember the goal: to lower and stabilize blood sugar levels. Read the Nutritional Facts on labels as shown previously. A low-sugar, low-carb diet typically focuses on the following food groups:

Proteins - Lean meats (such as chicken, turkey, and lean cuts of beef and pork), fish, seafood (including canned seafood in springwater or oil), eggs, and plant-based protein sources like tofu and tempeh. Aim on protein filling up "quarter of your plate".

Non-Starchy Vegetables - Vegetables that are low in carbohydrates and sugar, such as leafy greens (e.g., spinach, kale, lettuce), broccoli, cauliflower, zucchini, cucumbers, bell peppers, asparagus and pumpkin in moderation. Aim on these filling up "half of your plate".

Natural Healthy Fats - Sources of healthy fats with the least processing eg pasture raised meats and poultry, fatty fish eg Salmon, Sardines, Trout and Mackerel. Also avocados, olive oil, Ghee, coconut oil, nuts in moderation, and seeds e.g., chia seeds, sunflower, pepitas, flaxseeds. Aim on healthy fats filling up to "quarter of your plate".

Limited Low-Sugar Fruits (in limited moderation) - Berries e.g. strawberries, raspberries and small amounts of fruits like tomatoes and avocados. These fruits are relatively low in sugar compared to others. Refer to my Fruit & Vegetable lists.

Dairy - Full-fat dairy products like Greek yogurt, Tofu, plain yogurt, and low sugar cheese such as Mozzarella, but in moderation, as they contain some natural sugars (lactose).

Limited Legumes (in moderation) - Lentils, chickpeas, and black beans can be included in limited amounts as they provide protein and fiber but also contain carbohydrates.

Limited Grains - Whole grains like quinoa can be included in **very small quantities** for their fiber and nutrients, but portion control is important.

Beverages - Water, unsweetened herbal tea, and black coffee (without added sugar) are suitable beverages for a low-sugar, low-carb diet. Natural sweeteners such as Stevia, Xylitol and Monk Fruit may be added.

Nuts and Seeds (in moderation) - Nuts like almonds, walnuts, and seeds like chia and flaxseeds can be included in small portions for added healthy fats and fiber.

Salt, Herbs and Spices seasonings are allowed. They are a valuable addition as you tone down your taste buds.

6 Top Sugar Free Beverages

Water plays a crucial role in detoxification by aiding kidney and liver function, helping flush out toxins, and supporting overall bodily processes while following a no-sugar diet. No sugary drinks, however here are ideas.

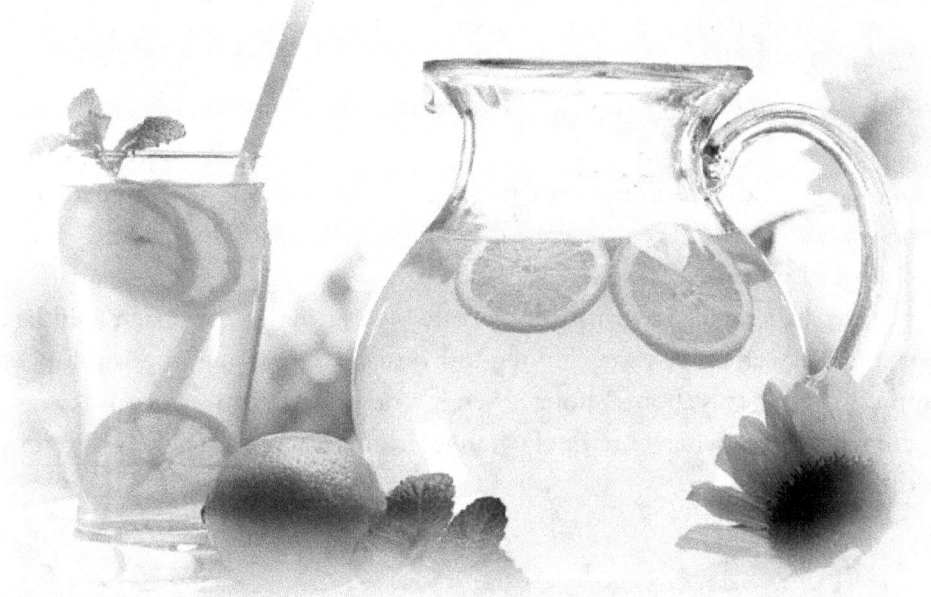

Suggested Beverages

Water - On its own, or with a slice of lemon or lime. Or a squeeze of lemon, lime or apple cider vinegar. Try adding a sprig of fresh mint if you have it in the garden.

Chia Water - Black chia seeds may help aid digestion and cleanse the stomach although evidence is not fully conclusive. They do help with satiety, or feeling full. But beware. Drink plenty of water with them as they absorb as much as 12 times their weight as they swell and become sticky. I only consume 1/2 tsp most days with water.

Teas & Coffee - Unsweetened tea, all herbal teas and black coffee. No sugar or honey. Ginger tea with freshly grated ginger. Peppermint tea can aid digestion.

Note about caffeine: Studies show our **cortisol levels (the stress hormone) peak early in the morning** to prepare for the day. That's why I avoid black coffee until late morning. Individuals may respond differently, so observe your anxiety/stress levels. Combining **high cortisol with caffeine can give an initial energy burst and anxiety, followed by an afternoon energy crash**.

Almond & Coconut Milk - Unsweetened almond milk typically contains 0-1 gram of sugar and 1-2 grams of carbohydrates per 1 cup serving.

Unsweetened coconut milk typically has a similar sugar and carbohydrate content, ranging from 0 to 1 gram of sugar and 1-2 grams of carbohydrates per 1 cup serving. Specific values may vary by brand.

If sweetening is necessary, use natural sweeteners such as; Stevia, Xylitol and Monk Fruit.

Notes: Avoid consuming caffeine (e.g., coffee or strong tea) immediately upon waking, as this may interfere with the natural cortisol rhythm and energy levels by causing an excess spike in cortisol.

In my experience, I drink black coffee on an empty stomach mid-late morning. This effect can vary among individuals, but for me, the window of suppressed hunger is about 2 hours, then it wears off... in time for consuming a late lunch. (This is when ghrelin, the hunger hormone, levels are likely to return to their baseline state.)

How Fats Stabilize Sugar Cravings

There is now supported and reputable research evidence from various trials and studies indicating that including dietary fat with a meal helps reduce post-meal glucose (sugar) spikes. This effect is particularly notable when the fat is healthy unsaturated fat.

Here are a few key points from research:

Satiety and Slower Digestion: Including healthy fats in a meal can increase feelings of fullness and satisfaction, which can lead to reduced overall food intake and a slower digestion process. This, in turn, can help stabilize blood sugar levels. Food combination is essential.

Improved Insulin Sensitivity: Some studies have shown that healthy fats, like those found in avocados, nuts, and olive oil, can improve insulin sensitivity, making it easier for the body to regulate blood sugar levels.

Balanced Meals: Meals that include a combination of macronutrients, including fats, carbohydrates, and proteins, tend to have a more moderate impact on blood sugar compared to high-carbohydrate meals.

Fiber and Fat: Meals that combine healthy fats with high-fiber foods, such as vegetables or whole grains, can be particularly effective in reducing blood sugar spikes.

Leptin, produced by fat cells, is a hormone that regulates appetite and energy balance. It signals the brain when the body has sufficient energy stores, reducing hunger and promoting a feeling of fullness. Leptin levels rise with increased fat mass and act to maintain body weight and energy balance.

Ghrelin is a hormone primarily produced in the stomach that stimulates hunger. It sends signals to the brain to increase food intake, leading to feelings of hunger.

Clinical trials have provided compelling evidence that dietary fat, especially when it's healthy and unsaturated, can have a profound impact on post-meal blood sugar levels. The slowing down of carbohydrate digestion and absorption by dietary fats contributes to a more stable and controlled response, effectively reducing the rapid spikes in blood glucose that often accompany high-carbohydrate meals.

Cream vs Milk - Surprising Facts

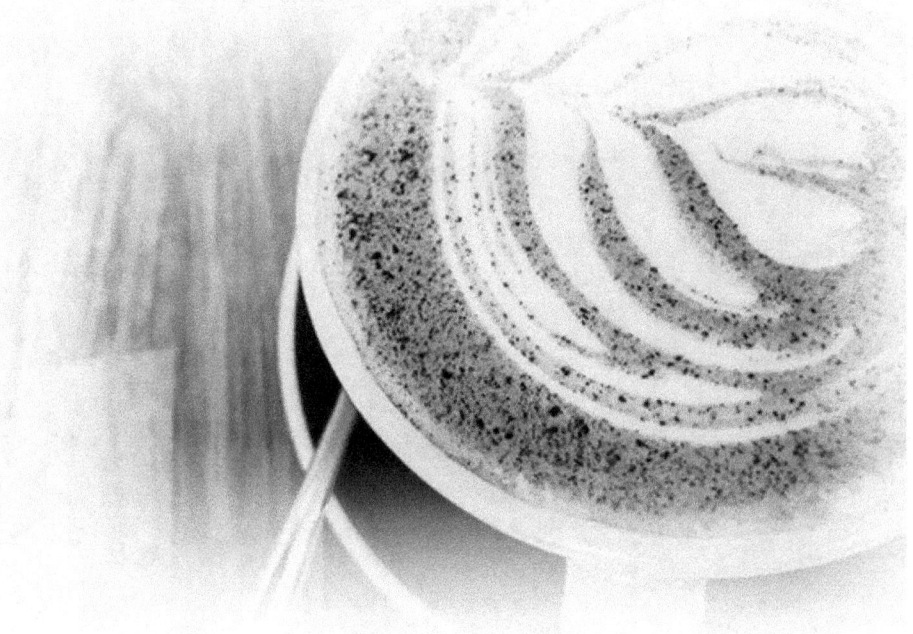

The difference between whole milk and heavy cream in terms of carbohydrates, sugars, lies in their fat content and water content. This is worth considering on a low sugar diet compared to a low fat diet.

Heavy/whole cream is a product with a very high fat content, typically around 36-40% fat by weight. **It contains minimal amounts of carbs and sugars**. The high fat content is why it's called "heavy" cream. Since it has very little water, there's less room for carbohydrates and sugars.

Whole milk contains a lower fat content than heavy cream, typically around 3.25-3.5% fat by weight. It also has a significant amount of water. **The carbs and sugars in whole milk come mostly from lactose, which is a naturally occurring sugar in milk**. The higher water content in milk dilutes the milk's other components, including the fat, protein, carbohydrates, and sugars.

So, when we compare whole milk to heavy cream, we find that **the presence of more water in whole milk means it can accommodate a higher amount of carbs and sugars per serving.** On the other hand, heavy cream, with its high fat content and lower water content, has very few carbohydrates and sugars.

Foods to Avoid for Sustained Success

A strict low-sugar and low-carb detox typically involves eliminating or significantly reducing the intake of foods and beverages that are high in sugar and carbohydrates. Here's a general list of items to eliminate. **You probably know of others you can add to the list yourself.**

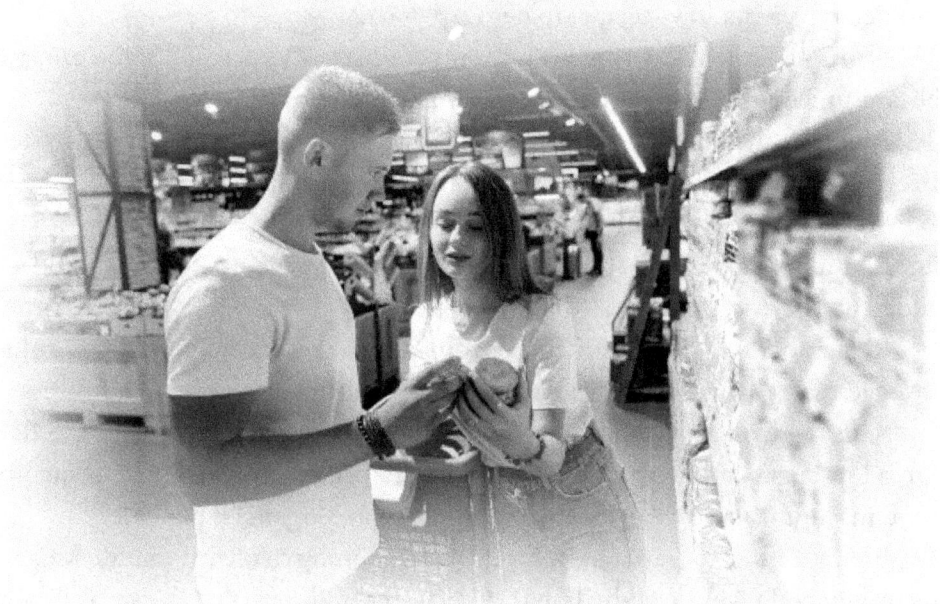

Strictly Avoid

Candy, Biscuits, Cakes, Breads and other sweets - These may be loaded with sugar and refined carbohydrates.

Flour-Based Products - This includes bread, pasta, pastries, and most baked goods, as they contain high levels of carbohydrates.

Dairy with Added Sugar - flavored yogurts, milkshakes, and certain processed dairy products that contain added sugar.

Sugar in All Forms - This includes table sugar, brown sugar, powdered sugar, and any other added sugar.

Starchy Vegetables such as potatoes and corn. Check the vegetables List and remove anything with a high carbohydrate content.

Sauces and Dressings - Many commercial sauces and salad dressings contain added sugar and hidden carbs. Opt for homemade or sugar-free alternatives. eg olive oil and Dijon mustard with egg yolk.

Sweeteners - This includes artificial sweeteners (like aspartame or sucralose) and natural sweeteners (honey, maple syrup, agave nectar, etc.) Opt instead for Stevia, Xylitol or Monk Fruit.

Dried Fruit - Dried fruits are concentrated sources of sugar and should be avoided on a strict low-sugar carb detox.

Fruits - While fruits are natural sources of sugar (fructose), some can still be consumed in moderation. Refer to my Detailed Fruit List.

Alcohol - Alcoholic beverages usually contain sugars or carbohydrates. Beer, wine, and cocktails plus others should all be eliminated.

Sugary Beverages - This includes all sugary drinks, such as soda, fruit juices, and energy drinks etc. Only Stevia, monk fruit or Xylitol should be added to hot drinks.

Remember - A glass of water first thing when you wake up in the morning is suggested. Add a lemon slice just for flavor or drink chia water.

Aim to drink around 8 glasses of water or similar throughout the day. On a low-sugar carb detox, focus on whole, unprocessed foods such as quality proteins, non-starchy vegetables, and healthy fats. Organic if possible.

It's important to learn about food labels carefully to identify hidden sugars in products. Staying well-hydrated with water and herbal teas can also help during the detox process.

How does exercise impact calories and energy burn?

This is applicable for those interested in weight loss. The actual number of calories burned during exercise will vary depending on factors like your weight, walking speed, and terrain. As a rough estimate you may find what Google says how much walking you need to do to get back to a "zero" calorie balance. Note some foods/beverages are negligible such as leafy greens and black tea or coffee.

1 Cup of Leafy Greens (e.g., spinach, kale, virtually calorie-free):

Leafy greens are extremely low in calories, so you likely won't need walking to offset the energy intake from 1 cup of leafy greens.

1 Cup of Black Tea or Coffee (virtually calorie-free if consumed without sugar or cream):

These beverages are very low in calories, so you may not need any additional walking to burn off the calories from a cup of unsweetened black tea or coffee.

1 Cup of Almond Milk (unsweetened, around 30 calories):

Approx. 5-10 minutes of brisk walking.

1 Cup of Unsweetened Coconut Milk (around 50 calories):

About 10-15 minutes of brisk walking.

1 Cup of Fresh Cooked Corn Kernels (around 130-150 calories, depending on preparation):

Approx. 25-35 minutes of brisk walking.

1 Apple (medium-sized, around 95 calories):

Approx. 20-30 minutes of brisk walking can burn off the calories in a medium-sized apple.

1 Slice of Wholemeal Bread (around 80-100 calories, depending on size and brand):

Approx. 15-25 minutes of brisk walking to burn off the calories in a slice of wholemeal bread.

Detailed Vegetable List by Ranking

Here's the list of common low sugar, low carb vegetables per 100 grams; including total carbohydrates, sugar content, glycemic index (GI - how quickly they convert into fuel and how long they keep you feeling full). Also included is fiber content and calories.

This includes both complex carbohydrates (starches) and simple carbohydrates (sugars). Spinach, zucchini, tomato, cauliflower, broccoli, green beans, kale, zucchini, bell peppers and onions are all heroes.

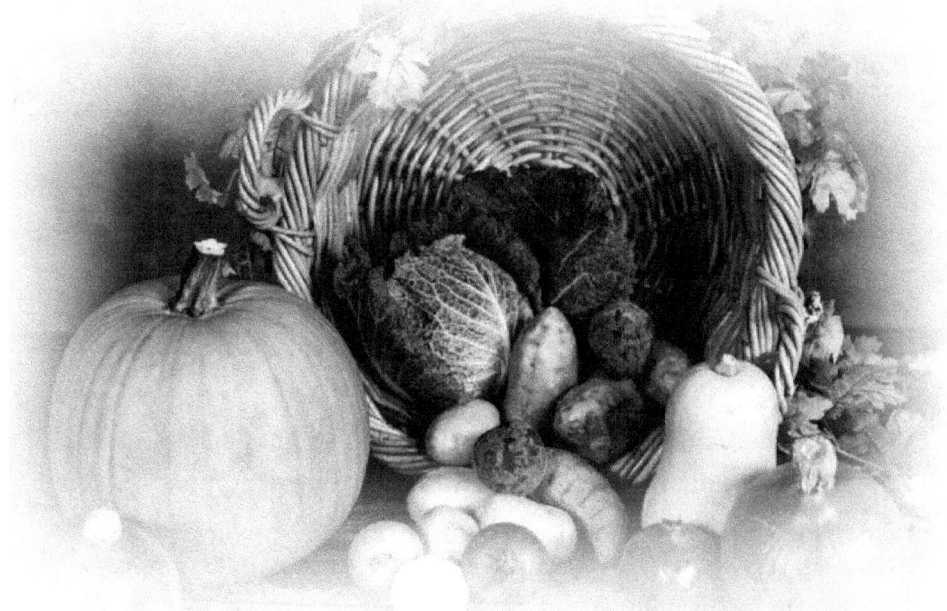

Avocado: Total Carbohydrates: Approx. 2 grams Sugars: Approx. 0.2 grams Glycemic Index (GI): Very low (estimated) Fiber: Approx. 6.7 grams Calories: Approx. 160 calories

Zucchini: Total Carbohydrates: Approx. 3.1 grams Sugars: Approx. 2.4 grams Glycemic Index (GI): Very low (estimated) Fiber: Approx. 1 gram Calories: Approx. 17 calories

Tomato, raw: Total Carbohydrates: Approx. 3.9 grams Sugars: Approx. 2.6 grams Glycemic Index (GI): Low (estimated) Fiber: Approx. 1.2 grams Calories: Approx. 18 calories

Spinach: Total Carbohydrates: Approx. 3.6 grams Sugars: Approx. 0.4 grams Glycemic Index (GI): Very low (estimated) Fiber: Approx. 2.2 grams Calories: Approx. 23 calories

Broccoli: Total Carbohydrates: Approx. 6.6 grams Sugars: Approx. 1.5 grams Glycemic Index (GI): Low (estimated) Fiber: Approx. 2.6 grams Calories: Approx. 55 calories

Cauliflower: Total Carbohydrates: Approx. 5 grams Sugars: Approx. 2 grams. Glycemic Index (GI): Low (estimated) Fiber: Approx. 2 grams Calories: Approx. 25 calories

Pumpkin: Total Carbohydrates: Approx. 7 grams Sugars:

Approx. 2.4 grams Dietary Fiber: Approx. 1 gram Calories: Approx. 20 calories

Kale: Total Carbohydrates: Approx. 8.7 grams Sugars: Approx. 2.3 grams Glycemic Index (GI): Low (estimated) Fiber: Approx. 2 grams Calories: Approx. 49 calories

Green Cabbage: Total Carbohydrates: Approx. 5.8 grams Sugars: Approx. 3.5 grams Glycemic Index (GI): Low (estimated) Fiber: Approx. 2.5 grams Calories: Approx. 25 calories

Green Beans: Total Carbohydrates: Approx. 6 grams Sugars: Approx. 3.3 grams. Glycemic Index (GI): Low (estimated) Fiber: Approx. 3.4 grams Calories: Approx. 31 calories

Bell Peppers, raw: Total Carbohydrates: Approx. 7-8 grams Sugars: Approx. 4-5 grams Protein: Approx. 1-2 grams Fat: Approx. 0-1 gram Fiber: Approx. 2-3 grams Total Calories: Approx. 31-32 calories

Red Cabbage: Total Carbohydrates: Approx. 7 grams Sugars: Approx. 3.8 grams Glycemic Index (GI): Low (estimated) Fiber: Approx. 2.1 grams Calories: Approx. 31 calories.

Avocado is one of my heroes! Higher in healthy fats, particularly monounsaturated fats, which contribute to its creamy texture. It's also rich in dietary fiber helping to promote feelings of fullness. In addition it is full of vitamins, minerals, and antioxidants making it a favorite indeed!

Retrogradation

The Glycemic Index (GI) measures how quickly carbohydrates in food are digested, affecting blood sugar levels. Lower GI foods can help manage diabetes and blood sugar. Cooking, cooling, and reheating can reduce the GI of certain starchy foods through a process called retrogradation.

Retrogradation involves starches forming a resistant structure after cooking and cooling, making them less digestible.

Studies suggest that starchy foods can have lower GIs when cooked, cooled, and reheated, due to the formation of resistant starch. However, the degree of GI reduction varies based on factors like starch type, cooling time, reheating method, and food preparation.

More research needs to be undertaken as studies show mixed results, with a 20-25% reduction in the GI of foods. Note, on a low carb diet rice and potatoes aren't recommended anyway.

Smoothies after detox?

After a sugar detox low sugar smoothies offer various health benefits. They are low in added sugars, as they primarily comprise fruits and vegetables, reducing overall sugar intake. Packed with nutrients, green smoothies contain leafy greens like kale and spinach, along with fruits and veggies, providing essential vitamins, minerals, and antioxidants.

Fiber is a significant component of green smoothies, aiding digestion, regulating blood sugar, and promoting satiety.

Hydration is also addressed, as recipes often include water, low sugar coconut water, almond milk etc. Green smoothies can be low in calories, making them a healthy snack or meal option that supports weight management. The antioxidants in green smoothies protect cells from free radical damage and may reduce the risk of chronic diseases.

Nutritional values of Fruits?

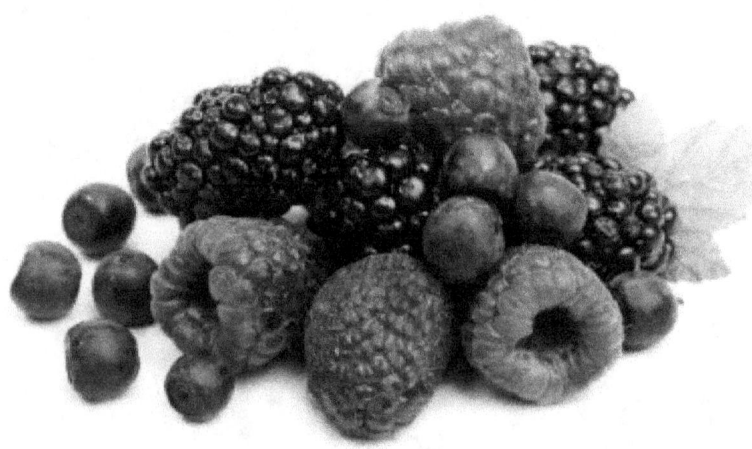

During the detox phase refrain from eating fruit all together with the exception being; lemons, limes, avocado, blackberries and strawberries. Only eat in strict moderation.

The following list of common low sugar fruits gives **Total carbs per 100 grams beginning from lowest (best) to highest the count.** If I eat low sugar fruit, it is at meal time, not as a snack due to the natural sugars spiking insulin. Low Glycemic Index (GI) fruits are best if you must.

Tomatoes (raw, average): Total Carbs: Approx. 4 grams Dietary Fiber: Approx. 1.2 grams Sugar: Approx. 3 grams Calories: Approx. 18 calories GI: Low (Approx. 15)

Cooked Rhubarb (no added sugar): Total Carbs: Approx. 4 grams Dietary Fiber: Approx. 1.7 grams Sugar: Approx. 1.7 grams Calories: Approx. 26 calories GI: Low (Approx. 15)

Lemons: Total Carbs: Approx. 9.3 grams Dietary Fiber: Approx. 2.8 grams Sugar: Approx. 2.5 grams Calories: Approx. 17 calories GI: Low (Approx. 20)

Limes: Total Carbs: Approx. 11 grams Dietary Fiber: Approx. 2.8 grams Sugar: Approx. 1.7 grams Calories: Approx. 30 calories GI: Low (Approx. 20)

Strawberries: Total Carbs: Approx. 8 grams Dietary Fiber: Approx. 3 grams Sugar: Approx. 4 grams Calories: Approx. 32 calories GI: Low (Approx. 40)

Cranberries: Total Carbs: Approx. 9.5 grams Dietary Fiber: Approx. 4.6 grams Sugar: Approx. 3.8 grams Calories: Approx. 46 calories GI: Low (Approx. 45)

Oranges: Total Carbs: Approx. 9 grams Dietary Fiber: Approx. 2.3 grams Sugar: Approx. 8.2 grams Calories: Approx. 43 calories GI: Medium (approx. 43)

Raspberries: Total Carbs: Approx. 9 grams Dietary Fiber: Approx. 8 grams Sugar: Approx. 2 grams Calories: Approx. 64 calories GI: Low (Approx. 32).

Blackberries: Total Carbs: Approx. 9 grams Dietary Fiber: Approx. 7 grams Sugar: Approx. 4 grams Calories: Approx. 40 calories GI: Low (Approx. 25)

Avocado: Total Carbs: Approx. 12 grams Dietary Fiber: Approx. 9 grams Sugar: Approx. 0.2 grams Calories: Approx. 160 calories GI: Low (Approx. 10)

Blueberries: Total Carbs: Approx. 14.5 grams Dietary Fiber: Approx. 2.1 grams Sugar: Approx. 9 grams Calories: Approx. 84 calories GI: Low (Approx. 53)

In comparison at the higher end of the carb content scale is;
Bananas: Approx. 22 grams of total carbohydrates.
Grapes: Approx. 18 grams of total carbohydrates.
Cherries: Approx. 16 grams of total carbohydrates.

Sugar Smart Tips to Achieve Your Goals

*Plan ahead so you don't waste food. Eat all perishable foods in the lead up to the start of the 7 day carb & sugar detox.

*Remove all alcohol and sugary, carb heavy foods from the pantry and fridge that you won't be using during the detox plan. Reduce temptation.

*"Listen" to your taste buds! If something tastes very sweet, it probably is. Your taste buds will learn to detect sugary foods and drinks as the days and weeks move forward.

*Foods advertised as "low fat" often have more sugar, so check labels. Refer to How to Read Food Labels.

Aim for high fibre, low sugar products but beware "lite" dairy products. During the 7 day sugar detox, it's best to eliminate all dairy. After this use unsweetened milks, unsweetened almond milk and coconut milk / coconut water in moderation.

*Don't eat fruit: During the detox phase don't eat any fruit (except lemons, limes, avocado, blackberries and strawberries in strict moderation.) **Most are moderate to high in natural sugars and carbs. Once detox is over**, you may add small portions of fruit on occasion. Fruit is full of fibre and nutrients, so it's acceptable not to eliminate it altogether.

*Avoid hidden sugar in dressings and sauces by reading labels. Replace store-bought options with homemade dressings using avocado, olive oil, lime juice or apple cider vinegar. Post-detox, include full-fat Greek yogurt for gut and brain health.

*To balance nutrition and beat hunger between meals, aim for your plate to be; 1/4 protein, 1/4 healthy fat and 1/2 vegetable/salad/seeds.

An example of the perfect no sugar no grain plate...

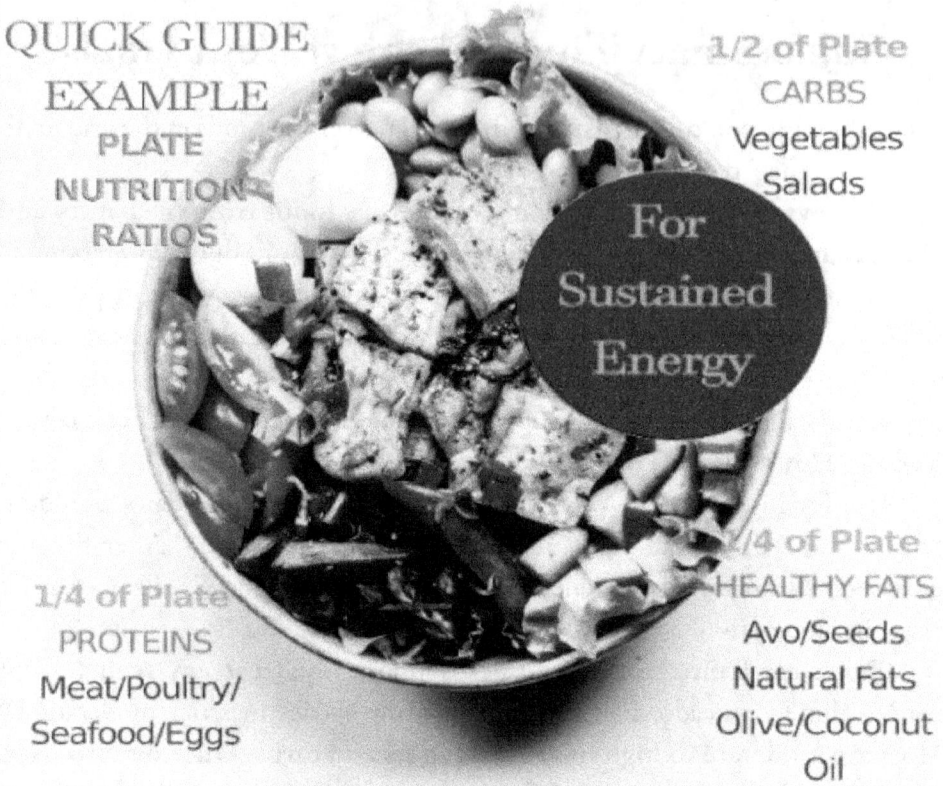

QUICK GUIDE EXAMPLE PLATE NUTRITION RATIOS

1/2 of Plate
CARBS
Vegetables
Salads

For Sustained Energy

1/4 of Plate
PROTEINS
Meat/Poultry/Seafood/Eggs

1/4 of Plate
HEALTHY FATS
Avo/Seeds
Natural Fats
Olive/Coconut Oil

Re Cholesterol: A sugar detox diet that includes an increase in healthy fats might have varying effects on cholesterol levels.

Healthy fats, such as those from avocados, nuts, fatty fish and olive oil, can be beneficial for heart health and help improve the balance of "good" (HDL) and "bad" (LDL) cholesterol. However, the overall impact on cholesterol depends on the volume, quality and specific fats consumed, dietary choices, and overall health. Talk with your GP.

In recent years, there has been a growing body of scientific research supporting the idea that the inclusion of dietary fats in our meals can help reduce post-meal glucose (sugar) spikes. This effect becomes particularly pronounced when those fats are of the healthy, unsaturated variety. Let's explore the evidence behind the glycemic control effect of dietary fat, shedding light on the potential benefits for our body, with particular attention to blood sugar regulation.

Prominent dietary patterns**, such as the Paleo diet, Mediterranean diet and more recently the Healthy Keto diet along with intermittent fasting, have been associated with improved glycemic control and a reduced risk of type 2 diabetes.**

Keto, low-sugar, and low-carb diets are all focused on restricting carbohydrate intake to varying degrees. The main points relating to all these dietary lifestyles are:

1. Keto diets are the most carb-restrictive, typically limiting carbs to under 50g per day to achieve a metabolic state of ketosis where the body burns fat for fuel instead of carbs.
2. Low-carb diets generally allow for a slightly higher carb intake, usually under 100-150g per day. This still prompts the body to burn more fat for energy while allowing for more carb-containing foods like vegetables and some fruits.
3. Low-sugar diets emphasize reducing added/refined sugars while carb intake can vary. This overlaps with keto and low-carb by cutting out sugary foods, desserts, sweetened beverages, etc.
4. All three diet approaches are intended to reduce inflammation by limiting carb-rich, processed foods that can contribute to inflammation. They emphasize whole, nutrient-dense foods like proteins, healthy fats, vegetables, etc.
5. Meal plans and recipes for keto, low-carb and low-sugar diets often overlap significantly, focusing on non-starchy vegetables, proteins, healthy fats, nuts/seeds, and low-sugar fruits.
6. The main distinction is the degree of carb restriction - keto being the most restrictive, low-carb allowing for more carbs from vegetables/fruits, and low-sugar diets moderating carbs while cutting added/refined sugars.

So in summary, Paleo, Keto, low-carb and low-sugar eating patterns are related in their emphasis on reducing carbs and sugars to varying extents, with the **goal of reducing inflammation, promoting fat-burning, and focusing on whole, unprocessed foods.**

Diets rich in healthy fats like those found in olive oil, nuts, and fatty fish when incorporated into a balanced diet, can help better manage blood sugar levels.

A reason I love using olive oil as a staple in my recipes, both raw and cooked. Suggested total carb count per meal on a sugar detox diet varies per individual, but is typically around 30-50 grams for women and 45-75 grams for men, emphasizing complex carbs from whole foods.

I began removing sugar and processed carbs from my diet over 5 years ago. Certain foods damage our immune system, negatively affect gut flora, weight gain and arthritis.

One key aspect of the glycemic control effect is the combination of dietary fiber and healthy fats. Foods like nuts, which contain both fiber and unsaturated fats, can effectively slow the absorption of carbohydrates, offering a double benefit in terms of blood sugar stabilization. **This combination is particularly powerful** in helping individuals manage their glucose response.

Healthy fats don't just influence blood sugar levels. They also have a positive effect on postprandial lipids, such as triglycerides and LDL cholesterol. Elevated levels of these lipids are risk factors for cardiovascular disease, and they can also be impacted by how our bodies regulate blood sugar.

In addition to their effect on glycemic control, some studies suggest that diets rich in healthy fats may improve insulin sensitivity. Enhanced insulin sensitivity is vital for blood sugar control, making this another reason to consider incorporating healthy fats into your low sugar meals.

In conclusion - The mounting evidence from various studies and reputable research supports the notion that dietary fats, especially healthy unsaturated fats, play a crucial role in glycemic control. This knowledge has significant implications for people seeking better blood sugar regulation and overall health.

It's important to remember a common sense approach that the specific outcomes may vary based on factors such as the type of fat consumed, the overall composition of the meal, and individual metabolic responses. As with any dietary guidance, it's advisable to consult with a healthcare professional or registered dietitian to receive personalized recommendations based on your unique health needs and goals.

Understanding the science behind the glycemic control effect of dietary fat empowers individuals to make informed dietary choices that can positively impact their well-being.

*Don't drink alcohol or fruit juices during the 7 day detox. Alcohol and juices have many hidden sugars and preservatives. Instead opt for lots of water, black herbal tea and coffee (in moderation)

*Consider breakfast.

Try eating a low GI healthy breakfast such as eggs accompanied with mushrooms, greens, bacon or tomato, avocado, bocconcini, a ham or bacon and egg bowl, an omelette or a healthy smoothie, or black chia seed pudding. Remember the nutritional balance to sustain energy.

***Always try to source fresh foods locally** and **buy organic** if possible. This reduces the possibility of pesticide residues from the plants and soils.

***Always wash fresh foods** before preparation.

Watch for unsuspected additives; **"Ingredients" on food labels; the largest quantity of an ingredient is typically listed first in the list.** Ingredients are listed in descending order of predominance by weight.

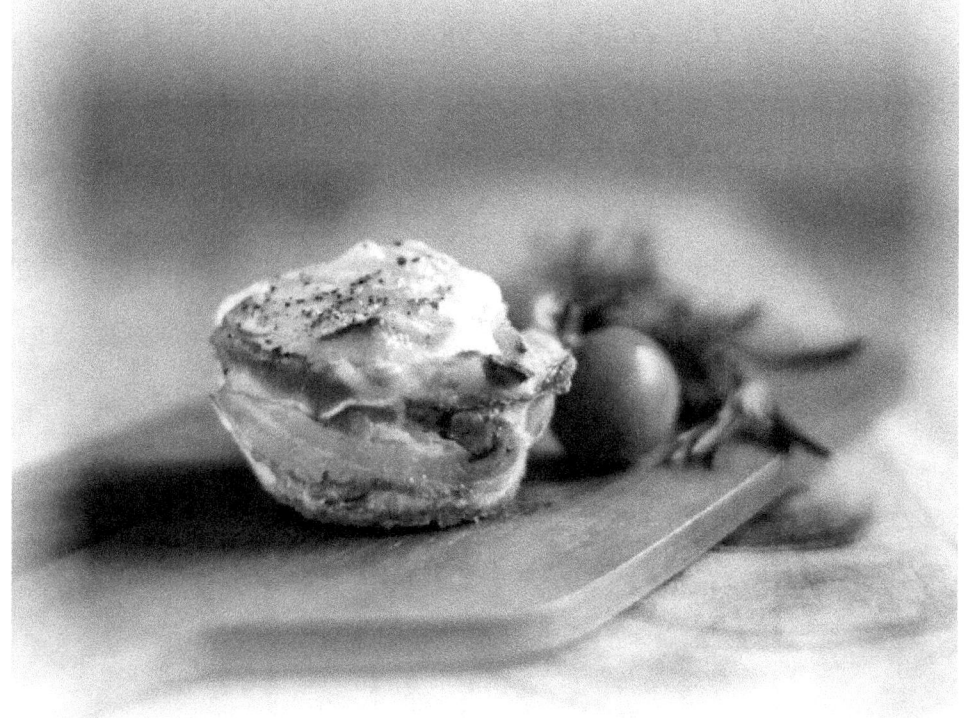

*Eggs are IN! Eggs are a low-carb and low-sugar food. In fact, they contain primarily healthy fats but virtually no carbohydrates or sugars. A large egg typically contains less than 1 gram of carbohydrates and less than 1 gram of sugar. Mostly composed of protein and healthy fats, eggs are a popular choice for following low-carb diets. The key vitamins found in eggs are amazing - Vitamin D, B12, A, E, K, B (B2, B5, B6, B9) and Choline.

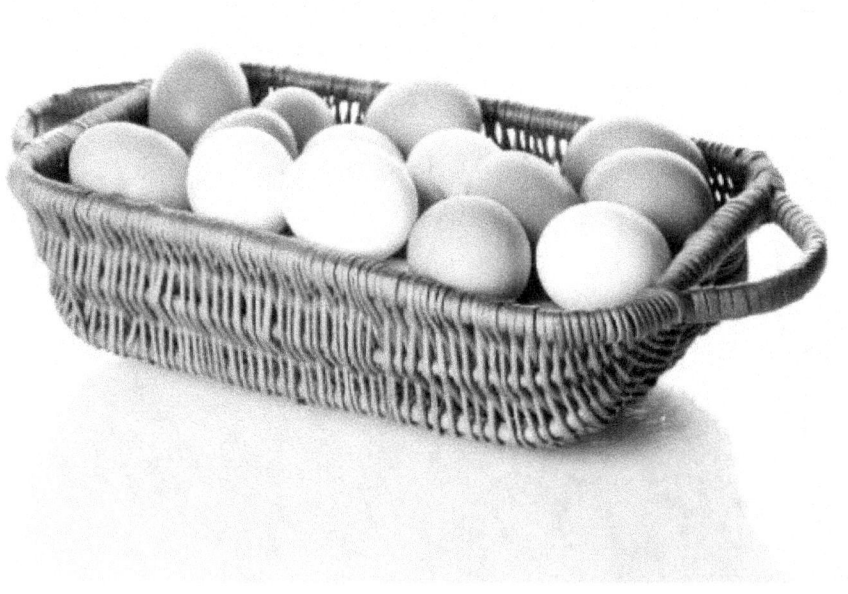

Depending on how you cook them, the yolk retains even more nutrition if you keep them soft. They are nature's little "nutrient packs" so eat these freely during detox. Consider raising some chickens in your own backyard! This is a wonderful way of recycling your food scraps and getting fresh organic eggs and free garden fertilizer in return!

My Iser Brown chickens...productive, happy proud girls indeed.

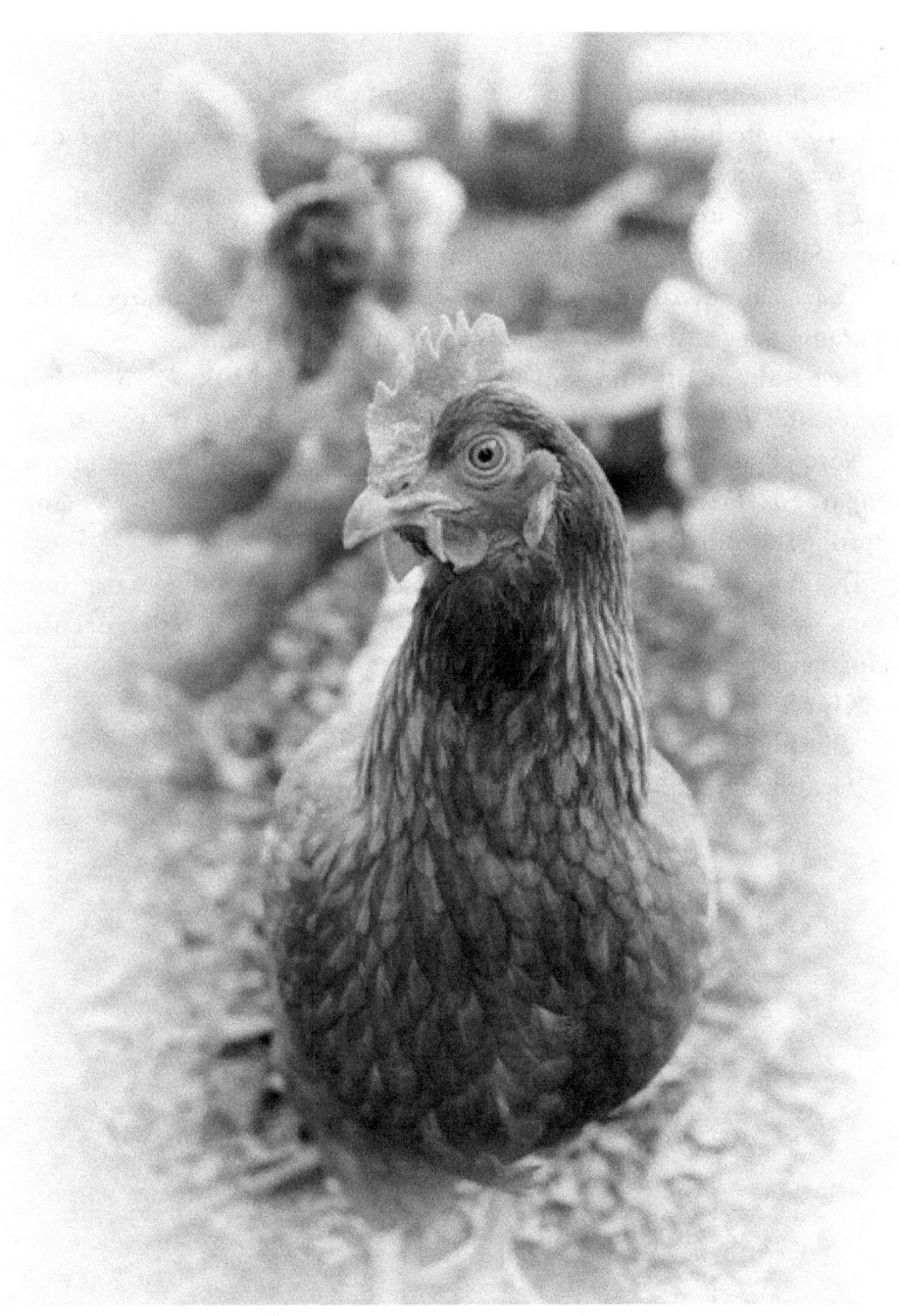

Cream or Milk?

Here's a comparison of the macronutrient content in 2 teaspoons of heavy cream compared with whole cow's and almond milk. (Generally low fat milks will have slightly higher carbs and less fat)

2 tsps/ about 10 grams of Heavy Cream: Carbohydrates: Approx. 0.4 grams. Sugar: Approx. 0 grams Fat: Approx. 7 grams

2 tsps / about 10 grams of Full/Whole Milk: Carbohydrates: Approx. 1.3 grams. Sugar: Approx. 1.3 grams Fat: Approx. 1.2 grams

2 tsp / about 10 grams of Unsweetened Almond Milk: Carbohydrates: Approx. 0.2 grams. Sugars: Less than 0.1 gram Fat: Approx. 0.2 grams

Note that whole milk contains more carbohydrates and sugar compared to heavy cream. This is because milk contains lactose, a naturally occurring sugar in dairy products.

Therefore adding a teaspoon of cream to your black coffee or tea (instead of milk) won't spike insulin. (Some people like to add a tsp of butter or coconut oil to their black coffee for this reason).

*Opt for Virgin Olive Oil or Coconut Oil.

*Opt for Organic products if possible.

*Health Supplements: Always take any medication as usual.

How to Quit Sugar & Beat Cravings

There are many good reasons to quit sugar. **Sugar can give us a short term energy boost. But it comes at a heavy price, often making us feel tired and moody... unless of course... we get more sugar, and thus creating the vicious cycle of sugar addiction.**

Retraining your taste buds pertains to the concept that by consistently consuming natural, whole foods with fewer additives and minimal processing, your taste preferences evolve. Over time, you'll discover an increased fondness for the flavors of fresh fruits, vegetables, whole grains, and other unprocessed foods, while your preference for highly processed, sugary, or artificially flavored foods diminishes. Interestingly, this phenomenon also applies to salt.

To develop healthier eating habits, we should retrain our taste buds to prefer natural foods and avoid processed packaged foods. This advice is grounded in the concept that our taste preferences can evolve based on our dietary

choices over time. (Personally, it took me about two weeks to 'retrain my body.' I no longer crave sugar and genuinely notice a significant difference in the taste of foods. My taste buds have been altered and retrained. Sugary foods now taste ...put simply...awful!)

Avoiding processed packaged foods is often recommended because they tend to be high in unhealthy ingredients like added sugars, artificial preservatives, and unhealthy fats.

Keep in mind that individual taste preferences can vary, and making dietary changes can be a gradual process. Some people may find it easier to transition to a healthier diet by making small, sustainable changes over time.

A 7-day food detox plan is a short-term dietary regimen designed to help cleanse the body, promote healthier eating habits, and potentially kickstart weight loss.

It will take about 5 - 7 days to rid your body of hidden sugars. If you experience withdrawal symptoms in the initial stages of sugar detox, including cravings, mood swings, and headaches. These

symptoms typically subside within a week or so. Stay strong.

Preparing for 7 days of Healthy Eating

Inventory in fridge and pantry. If you have lots of fruit for example, you may want to start the detox plan after using up fresh foods so they don't go to waste. Initially you may want to remove any undesired "temptation" foods.

Stock up on the 7 Day Low Carb/Sugar Foods

Go shopping. Stock up on your essential items in preparation for the detox phase. Look at recipes. Buy plenty of low sugar vegetables, greens and meats, canned fish, fresh fish, avos, for salads, seeds, nuts, spices, herbs etc. Buy limited tofu, lentils. Buy unsalted nuts, oils, chia seeds and other ingredients for the recipes you want to use. Eat unlimited eggs and non starchy veggies as suggested.

NOTES

Print planners reminder, write down items to stock your pantry

Drink Plenty of Water

Remove all drinks from your diet that have sugar in them during the detox phase; Juices, sodas, hot sugary beverages and alcohol. Did you know that water not only hydrates our body but also helps dilute and flush out toxins? This is wonderful when trying to detox your body of excess salts and sugars in the bloodstream. You will urinate more often and your stomach will feel better too. Start with a glass of water first thing each morning to get your kidneys active. Similarly, drinking black herbal or black coffee with no sugar or milk is okay. Try adding some lemon for a twist. It's refreshing and great for weight loss.

A Note About Caffeine and Cortisol

Studies show our cortisol levels (the stress hormone) peak early in the morning to prepare for the day. That's why **I avoid drinking my black coffee until mid-late morning**. Individuals may respond differently, so observe your anxiety/stress /energy levels. Combining high cortisol with caffeine can give an initial energy burst and anxiety, however followed by an afternoon energy crash.

Eat Low Sugar Vegetables

Eat at least 5 servings of vegetables per day that are low in sugars. Refer to the vegetable list. Remove the starchy varieties such as potatoes, peas and corn. Try to half fill your plate with suggested vegetables on the list.

Eat Healthy Foods

Foods with high protein and healthy fats such as eggs, nuts, natural meats and tofu, lentils, and bean sprouts are great for satisfying hunger and giving energy. Vegetables with complex carbohydrates keep you satiated for much longer. Some are strictly limited as per recipes.

Eat Regularly

One of your main goals when quitting sugar is keeping yourself satisfied with foods and keep your metabolism kicking along. If you skip meals, it is more likely that you would give into temptation of getting a quick sugar boost. It is easier to control what you eat, if you do it every three to five hours. This strategy will keep your blood sugar stable. Don't try starving yourself...your body will win.

Read Sugar Content on Labels

Manufacturers add sugar and other nasty chemicals to many products, often in unexpected products. For example, almost all ketchup brands contain sugar. Many reduced-fat products make up for the lack of fat with added sugar.

When reading a label on a food item, **pay attention to the different types of sugars like corn syrup, brown sugar, maple syrup, etc**. Manufacturers can avoid listing sugar as one of the main ingredients. Beware corn syrup, dextrose and honey (although honey is at least natural)

The Low Sugar Low Fat Myth

Common Myth:
"Low-fat foods are healthy and help me to lose weight."

The Reality: Our bodies, especially the brain, require healthy fats for optimal function and to curb sugar cravings. Many low-fat or reduced-fat foods compensate for the loss of flavor and texture when fat is removed by adding carbs and sugars. **People often choose these foods, thinking they are making a healthier choice, but, in reality they might be consuming excess sugar and calories.**

Monitoring Labels for Culprits - Many processed foods labeled as "low-fat" may contain added sugars to compensate for the reduced fat content. Here are some examples of processed foods that can be low in fat but high in sugar per gram:

LOW FAT VANILLA FLAVOURED YOGHURT
INGREDIENTS: Skim **Milk**, Concentrated Skim **Milk**, Water, Sugar, Cream (From **Milk**), Thickeners (1422 (From Maize), 1442 (From Maize)), **Milk** Solids, Gelatine, Flavours, Acidity Regulators (331, 332, 270, 330), Enzyme (Lactase), Live Cultures.
Contains Milk and Milk Products.

*Flavored Yogurt & Ice Cream - Low-fat or fat free yogurt is often sweetened with added sugars to enhance its taste. Fruit-flavored yogurts, in particular, can be high in sugar.

*Breakfast Cereals - Certain breakfast cereals, especially those marketed as low-fat cereals, may contain added sugars, or be carb dense to make up for the lack of fat.

*Fat-Free Salad Dressings and Spreads - Some fat-free salad dressings can have a higher sugar content to enhance flavor and texture.

*Low-Fat Baked Foods such as cookies, savoury biscuits, muffins, and other baked goods that are labeled as low-fat often have additional sugar to make up for the reduced fat content.

*Fruit Snacks and Desserts - Packaged fruit snacks marketed as low-fat or fat-free may have added sugars to improve taste and shelf life.

*Low-Fat Snack Bars - Certain low-fat or diet snack bars may contain high levels of sugars, such as fructose, glucose, or syrups, to enhance flavor and texture.

As you can see, it's essential to read food labels and check the nutritional information per 100gm

*Fruit Snacks and Desserts - Packaged fruit snacks marketed as low-fat or fat-free may have added sugars to improve taste and shelf life.

*Low-Fat Snack Bars - Certain low-fat or diet snack bars may contain high levels of sugars, such as fructose, glucose, or syrups, to enhance flavor and texture.

As you can see, it's essential to read food labels and check the nutritional information per 100gm.

Remember, low-fat foods with added sugars and high carbs can lead to immediate unexpected issues including insulin spikes and increased hunger.

*Calorie Intake: If fat is reduced in a product, but sugars are added for flavor, the overall calorie content may not be significantly lower. This can lead to over consumption of calories.

*Blood Sugar Spikes: Added sugars can cause rapid spikes in blood sugar levels, which are not conducive to maintaining steady energy levels and can lead to overeating.

*Sugar Dependency: Regular consumption of low-fat, high-sugar foods can lead to sugar cravings and dependency.

*Weight Gain: Consuming more calories than your body needs, whether from sugars or other sources, can contribute to weight gain.

To make informed food choices, it's essential to read food labels and understand the ingredients used in low-fat products. Look for products that have limited or no added sugars and focus on the overall nutritional profile rather than just the fat content.

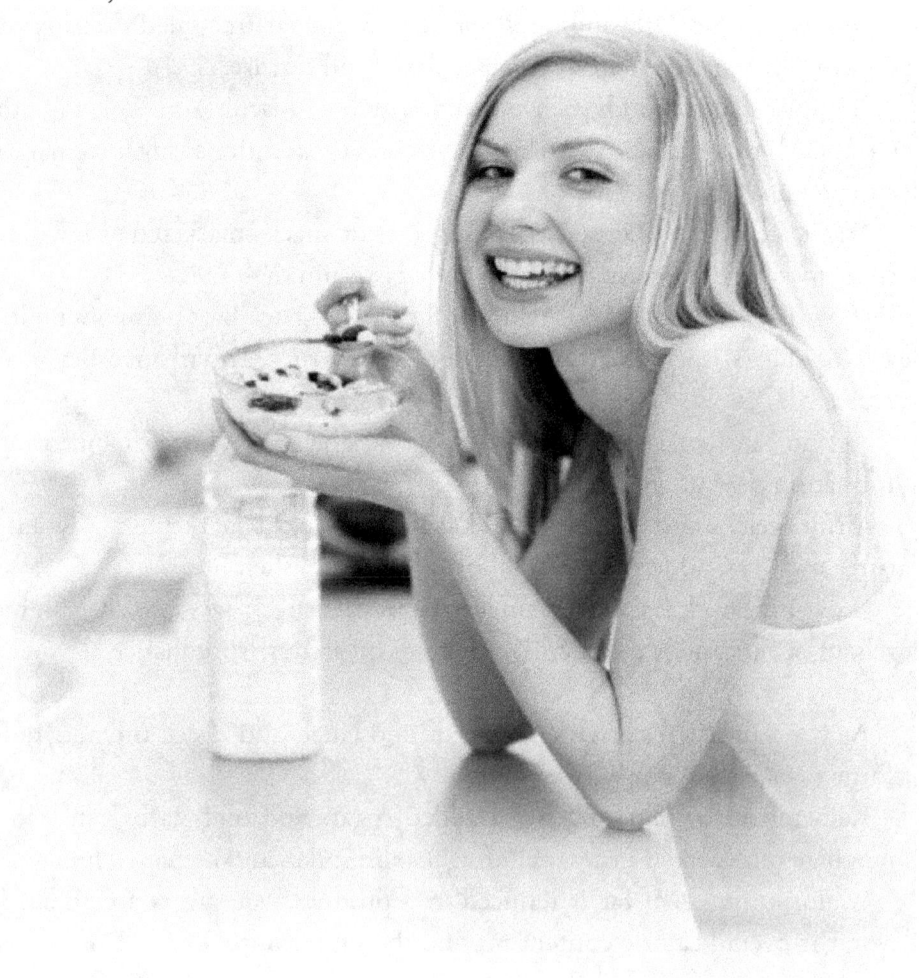

Notice the Pattern?
Note... **the main culprits are the processed foods.**

Ignore big brand advertising displayed on the front of the box if it seems misleading! Instead, **take an in-depth look at the food labels listing nutritional breakdown yourself.** Also, inspect the ingredients closely. Just another good reason to eat a clean diet with unadulterated whole foods without hidden ingredients.

This screenshot from WebMD:

When you read the labels on foods in your supermarket, it's no surprise that you find plenty of sugar in products like cake mix, ice cream, jelly, cookies, and soda. But it ca be downright shocking to see 12 grams of sugar in bottled pasta sauce or barbecue sauce -- and even more so to find 50 grams of sugar in a healthy-sounding bottled tea

To help you ferret out which products are surprisingly high in sugar, I embarked on a mission in the aisles of my local market. Over the course of several days, with my reading glasses close at hand, I examined hundreds of nutrition information labels to check out the sugar content in foods.

One thing's for sure: Just because there's a nutrition-oriented statement on the package (like "contains whole grain," "excellent source of calcium," "fat-free," "100% juice" or "25% less sugar") doesn't mean it *doesn't* contain a shocking amount of sugar. And just because the brand name or product name sounds like it's good for weight loss (Weight Watchers, Skinny Cow, etc.), don't assume the food is lower in sugar.

So how much exactly is a gram of sugar? One teaspoon of granulated sugar equals 4 grams of sugar. To put it another way, 16 grams of sugar in a product is equal to abou 4 teaspoons of granulated sugar.

Keep in mind, though, that the grams of sugar listed on the nutrition information label includes natural sugars from fruit (fructose) and milk (lactose) as well as added sweeteners like refined sugar or high-fructose corn syrup. That's why the label on a carton of regular low-fat milk says there's 13 grams of sugar per cup. And that's why the grams of sugar per serving in Raisin Bran (or any cereal with raisins or other drie fruit) seem unexpectedly high.

Complex Carb Count in Common Foods

A Quick Look at Potato, Rice, Lentils & Quinoa

Look at this comparison giving approximate counts for carbohydrate and sugar content per 100 grams for lentils, potatoes, rice, and quinoa. They will be strictly limited.

Lentils (Cooked)

Total Carbohydrates: Approx. 20 grams Sugars: Approx. 2 grams. Lentils are low in sugar and provide complex carbohydrates, fiber, and protein, making them a nutritious choice.

White Potato (Boiled, without skin)

Total Carbohydrates: Approx. 20 grams Sugars: Approx. 1 gram. White potatoes are moderate in carbohydrates and have low sugar content.

White Rice (Cooked)

Total Carbohydrates: Approx. 28 grams Sugars: Approx. 0 grams. White rice is higher in carbohydrates but has no naturally occurring sugars.

Quinoa (Cooked)

Total Carbohydrates: Approx. 21 grams Sugars: Approx. 1.6 grams. Quinoa is a pseudograin that contains complex carbohydrates and small amounts of natural sugars.

In summary, lentils and white potatoes have similar carb content per 100 grams, with lentils having slightly more fiber. White rice is higher in carbohydrates compared to the other options but contains no natural sugars. Quinoa falls between lentils and rice in terms of carb content, with a small amount of natural sugars. As complex carbs they should be used in strict moderation.

Low-Carb Breads: Read labels. Truly **low-carb breads** typically contain under 10g total carbs per serving (1-2 slices). Therefore eat in strict moderation.

Total Carbs or Net Carbs?

Regarding the basics of a low sugar diet, this info on the difference in carbs and net carbs may interest you. **Net carbs take into account the fiber in a food item**. The calculation for net carbs involves subtracting the grams of dietary fiber and certain sugar alcohols (like erythritol) from the total carbohydrates.

Dietary fiber is not fully absorbed and metabolized by the body, and therefore has minimal impact on blood sugar levels. Sugar alcohols also have a limited effect on blood sugar, and they are often subtracted from total carbs when calculating net carbs. (That's why celery is good).

By subtracting fiber and these specific sugar alcohols, you **get the net carb value, which is used as a measure of the carbohydrates that have a more significant impact on blood sugar in the context of low-carb diet plans**. We are aiming for a balanced natural food diet low to very low in carbohydrates, typically containing around 40-60 grams of carbs per day depending on each individual. After detox this may be increased to a maximum of around 100. But if we take the net carbs into consideration, the real impact on our sugar levels would be more accurate.

The calculation is as follows:
Net Carbs = Total Carbs – Fiber
You may apply this equation to all recipes.

Example - 1 cup (about 89 grams) of raw cabbage has Approx. 5.8 grams of total carbs and 2.2 grams of fiber.

The equation for net carbs is:
Net Carbs = Total Carbs (5.8) – Fiber (2.2)
Net Carbs = 5.8 gram – 2.2 grams
Net Carbs ≈ 3.6 grams

How to Control Carb Detox Side Effects

The Good

Here are some of the beneficial side effects associated with reducing or eliminating added sugars from your diet:

Stabilized Blood Sugar - A sugar detox can help regulate blood sugar levels, reducing the risk of blood sugar spikes and crashes.

Reduced Sugar/Carb Cravings - Over time, you'll likely experience fewer sugar cravings, making it easier to resist sugary foods.

Weight Management - Reducing added sugars can contribute to weight loss and help maintain a healthy weight.

Improved Energy Levels - Many people report increased and more consistent energy levels without the fluctuations caused by sugar intake.

Better Skin Health - Lower sugar intake may lead to improved skin health, with fewer breakouts and a more radiant complexion.

Better Mood - Stable blood sugar levels can lead to improved mood and reduced mood swings.

Better Oral Health - Reducing sugar intake can have a positive impact on oral health, reducing the risk of cavities and gum disease.

Improved Heart Health - Lower sugar intake is associated with reduced risk factors for heart disease, such as lower blood pressure and improved cholesterol levels.

Reduced Inflammation - Lower sugar consumption may lead to reduced inflammation in the body, which is associated with various chronic health conditions.

Enhanced Taste Perception - Over time, you may find that your taste buds become more sensitive, allowing you to appreciate the natural flavors of food.

Better Sleep - Some people experience improved sleep quality after reducing sugar intake.

The Not So Good

We are all different and while you will benefit from most of the "Good Side Effects" you may only need to endure some of the "Not So Good" side effects for a few days if at all.

Sugar Cravings - One of the most common side effects is intense cravings for sugary and carb heavy foods, especially in the first few days.

Headaches - Some people experience headaches, often due to the drop in blood sugar levels.

Mood Swings - You may experience mood swings, irritability, or mood fluctuations as your body adapts.

Fatigue - A decrease in sugar intake can initially lead to feelings of fatigue and low energy.

Digestive Issues - Changes in your diet may temporarily affect your digestion, leading to issues like bloating, gas, or diarrhea.

Sleep Disturbances - Some people report sleep disturbances or difficulty falling asleep during the initial stages.

Lightheadedness - A drop in blood sugar levels can cause lightheadedness or dizziness.

Muscle Aches - You may experience muscle aches and pains, similar to flu-like symptoms.

Crash in Energy - After the initial sugar rush, you might experience a drop in energy levels.

Reduced Focus and Concentration - Some people find it difficult to focus during the initial stages of a sugar detox.

It's important to note that these side effects are usually temporary and vary in intensity from person to person. They typically subside within a few days to a couple of weeks as your body adjusts to lower sugar intake. Staying well-hydrated, eating balanced meals, and getting plenty of rest can help alleviate some of these side effects.

Many find that by removing toxins from the body such as sugars, processed foods, preservatives, artificial flavours and colours will help them feel better quickly because you won't be in a "thought fog". Digestion and sleep quality are often better too. Many people will find you won't need as much sleep. (I did).

The label below on a processed food package is a classic example of foods with added ingredients detrimental to our health such as the varieties of sugars, molasses corn syrup, hydrogenated oils, artificial flavours...the list goes on. Side effects can vary, but this is only flour!

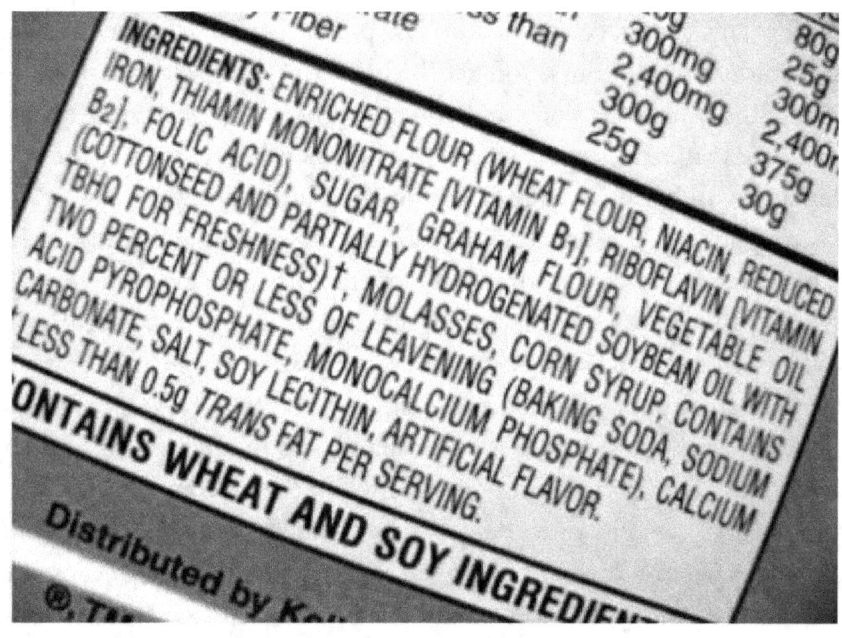

In Summary - The benefits of removing sugar and following a low carbohydrate diet are many. A short term adjustment for a long term achievement.

7 Day Low Carb Meals (No Calorie Counting)

Before we begin, let's start with a basic overview. The 7-day set of recipes is to guide you on your sugar-free detox journey. **During this stage, it's essential to completely eliminate processed sugar in all forms, including beverages, and focus on recommended foods.** This means consuming foods with no added sugar and those that are naturally low in sugars. When transitioning to a low-carb diet, your body goes through an adjustment period.

Please read labels when you shop. In addition to omitting sugars, don't buy or use any products with additives, preservatives, artificial sweeteners, artificial colours and flavours. You get the idea...the goal is clean, natural eating to clear toxins from your body. Natural sweeteners suggested may be used in moderation as an early sugar replacement. **Remember, as you eat less carbs and sugar, it will be easier to break your sugar addiction.**

If struggling on the first few days and want to snack, consider drinking water, black tea or coffee, eat some leafy greens with a drizzle of olive oil, or go for a walk. (This works for me; 1 long black weak coffee mid morning and 1 mid afternoon) Your body's main fuel source was carbs before, now cravings are hormonal fluctuations as your body adjusts.

Hunger pangs come in waves and usually pass in about 10 mins. Staying well-hydrated. Eating balanced meals with the recommended mix of macronutrients, which include protein, small portions of complex carbohydrates (eg firm tofu (0.5g), boiled soybeans (2.4g), mung beans (11.6g), and fat, can help mitigate most, if not all, of these effects. **Don't skimp on macros, including protein and fat.** The first few days often pose the biggest challenge. If you previously consumed lots of sugar and experience a headache, take your usual pain relievers if necessary to help you get through. Expect some minor hurdles.

Here's a breakdown of the points

Cravings and Withdrawal - It is not uncommon for individuals transitioning from a high-carb, high-sugar diet to experience cravings and withdrawal symptoms as the body adjusts to reduced carbohydrate intake.

Stay focused on the rewards, I found the symptoms were replaced by feeling amazing!

Recipe Adjustment - Increasing the volume (calories) of the low-carb recipes initially can be a strategy to help manage cravings. This approach may work for some individuals, but the degree of adjustment needed can vary from person to person.

Headaches and "Low Carb Flu" - Some people may experience symptoms often referred to as "low-carb flu," which can include headaches and fatigue. Staying hydrated and ensuring sufficient electrolyte intake can help alleviate these symptoms in most cases. Be patient as your body adjusts.

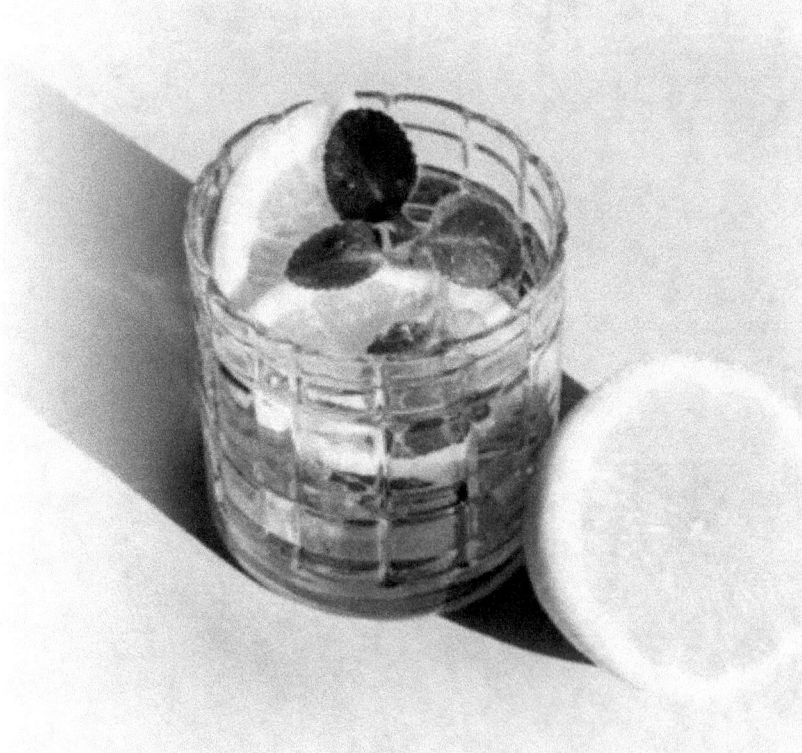

Balanced Nutrition - Consuming a balanced combination of carbohydrates, protein, and fats is essential for overall health and to help reduce cravings. This balanced approach can also help stabilize blood sugar levels.

Individual Variation - Every individual's response to dietary changes is unique. Some may adapt more smoothly, while others may require a longer adjustment period. If this is you, simply repeat and continue.

*If you want to change cooking methods or add extra low carb vegetables to ANY of the meals feel free to do so!

Recipes Optional Extras: You may see optional extra ingredients during some recipes. There is no limit on low carb vegetables & salads. But, also remember the important role of protein and fats for energy.

*If you get hungry before your "usual" dinner time, feel free to eat early. For better digestion, eating 2 hours before bedtime is recommended. A short walk or light exercise after dinner will help digestion, help regulate blood sugar levels and aid weight loss.

The nutrient breakdown provided is for the entire recipe as everybody's lifestyle and needs are different.

*Consume any leftovers the next day or freeze as applicable.

***Recipes are flexible.** You're learning about an easy low carb dietary change, **not being a slave to exact calorie counting. You do not want to be hungry!**

*For adaptability, adjust the recipe to your individual needs without stressing over precise amounts. It's a great way to empower you to make the dish work for you. To help guide you - **the nutritional breakdown provided** (carbs, sugars, protein, fat, fiber, and calories) **that are for the entire recipe,** so divide this by the number of servings you will get out of each recipe. Serving sizes are suggested.

Portion sizes?

Individual nutritional needs vary such as age, gender, activity level, your personal dietary goals, and for those with specific health conditions. Due to this accuracy varies. Consult with a registered dietitian or healthcare professional.

Nutrients per Recipe

But, if you have the total nutritional breakdown for the entire recipe, you can determine the nutritional content per serving by dividing those values by the number of servings based on your needs.

The formula for calculating the nutritional content per serving is:

$$\text{Nutrient per Serving} = \frac{\text{Total Nutrient in Recipe}}{\text{Number of Servings}}$$

For example, if you have a recipe that makes four servings, and you eat it in four servings, you would divide the total nutrient values (carbs, sugars, protein, fat) by four to get the nutrient content per serving. This allows you to have a more accurate representation of the nutritional information for a single serving size.

Keep in mind that the actual serving size may vary, so it's essential to consider how the recipe is portioned and adjust the calculations accordingly.

No need to be exact with measurements; the recipes are designed for easy flexibility to fit into your serving size needs to ensure your success. Don't lose sight of the overall goal.

Be strong. If you falter one day, pick it up the next. I, like many others, have been there. Gradually your body will adapt to fewer carbs.

Celery snacks. The nutritional content of 1/2 cup (about 50 grams) of raw celery is Approx. Calories: 6, Total Carbohydrates: 1.2 gr, Fiber: 0.6 gr, Sugars: 0.6 gr, Protein: 0.3 gr, Fat: 0.1 gr. Negligible amounts make it a perfect snack and have little impact on sugar spikes.

Enjoy the journey to a new better sugar free You!

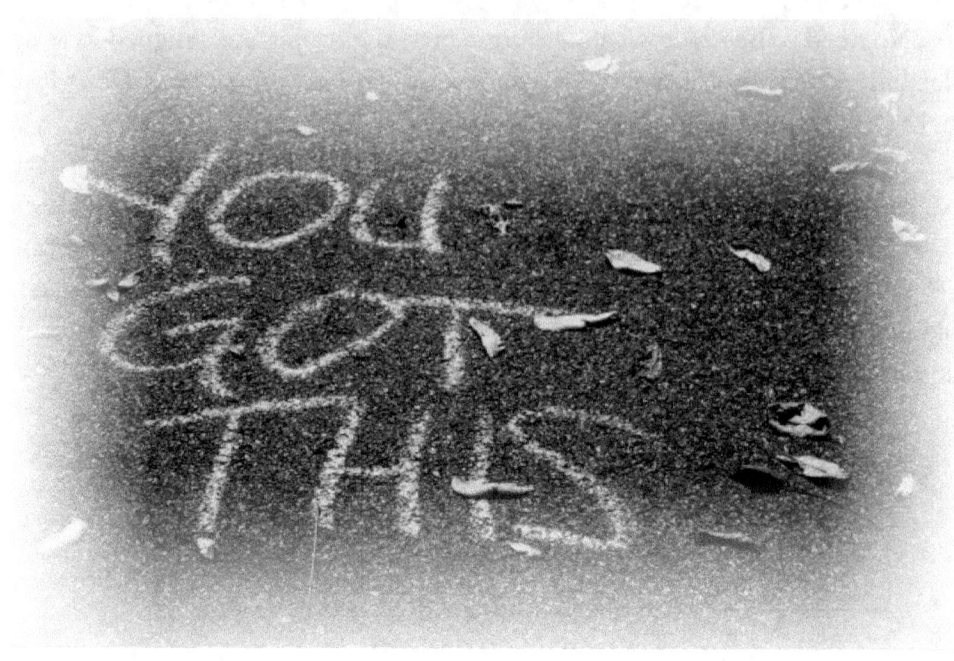

Day 1

Before Breakfast: A Glass of Water

Breakfast: Hard Boiled Eggs & Detox Smoothie

Lunch: Fresh Shrimp Seafood Salad & Chia Seed Water

Dinner: Crumbed Cashew Chicken & Garden Salad

Beverages: Water, Herbal Black Tea or Coffee (coffee suggested from late morning)

Snack: Celery & Natural Peanut Butter

Nutritional Breakdown is Per Recipe (Carbs, Sugars, Protein, Fat, Fiber and Calories.) Divide by your serving size

Net Carbs = Total Carbs – Fiber

Notes: I drink a long black coffee or tea mid-late morning and sometimes mid afternoon. Personal choice. I like it and it curbs my appetite. Cortisol, our natural stress hormone that peaks in the morning hours, should not be further elevated by consuming caffeine from coffee or strong tea immediately upon waking, as this may interfere with the body's natural cortisol rhythm and energy levels.

Occasionally I add 1 tsp whole cream. Zero sugars. Try it!

Celery Snacks: The perfect snack at 1.2 gm of total carbs for 1/2 cup. Eat if still feeling hungry (or juice it). Preferably eat celery on its own, or with a small amount of peanut butter or Tofu. Beware peanut paste with added sugars. Read the labels. Source organic if possible with nothing else added but peanuts.

For dinner you get to choose a large salad and/or vegetables from the suggested detailed vegetable list. This is always good when you have things in the fridge you want to use up and not waste.

Hard Boiled Eggs

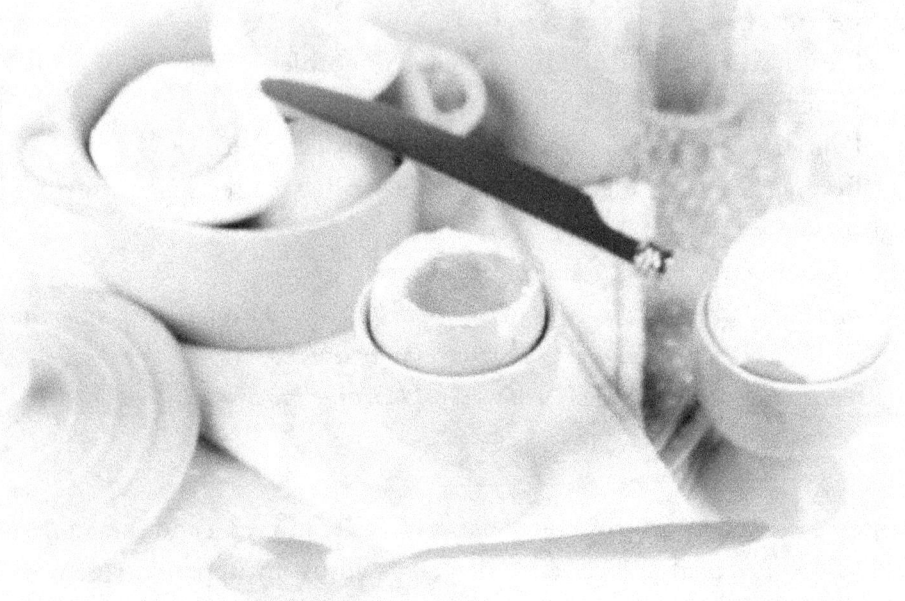

We don't want fancy or difficult recipes, we just want sustainable nutritious low sugar foods! The humble egg provides just that. Fabulous for detox and a no sugar diet. With <1 gram of carbs and sugar it simply can't be overlooked. An egg typically contains 6 g of protein, 5 g of fat, negligible carbs. One of our food staple favorites. It's versatile, straight from nature and consisting of a good protein, fat and vitamin balance.

Serving size 1 |

Ingredients:

1 - 2 fresh eggs

Place water in small saucepan with lid a pinch of salt (makes peeling easier)

Directions: If eggs are room temperature use tap water, if cold use cold water - so they don't crack.

Place the fresh eggs gently in an empty saucepan.

1. Fill the pot with enough water to completely cover eggs. Turn heat on to high and bring eggs to the boil.
2. Turn to low, simmer for another 3 - 5 minutes depending if you like soft or hard boiled eggs.

To help, take an egg out & spin it on the bench. (If it spins quickly it's more hard boiled than if it spins slowly) 3. Once done, plunge into cold water under a running tap and peel.

Total Carbohydrates for Recipe: Less than 1 gram Sugars: Negligible

Protein: 6 grams Fat: 5 grams Fiber: Negligible Total Calories: 120-150 (depending on egg size)

Notes: Eggs contain minimal carbs, are a rich source of high-quality protein and healthy fats. The sugar content is due to naturally occurring sugars, primarily in the form of glucose and fructose. Eggs are also a source of essential vitamins and minerals, making them a nutritious addition to a balanced diet. If you have your own backyard free range chickens, their eggs will hold even more nutrients due to the added grubs, worms, grasses and weeds they eat!

Detox Smoothie

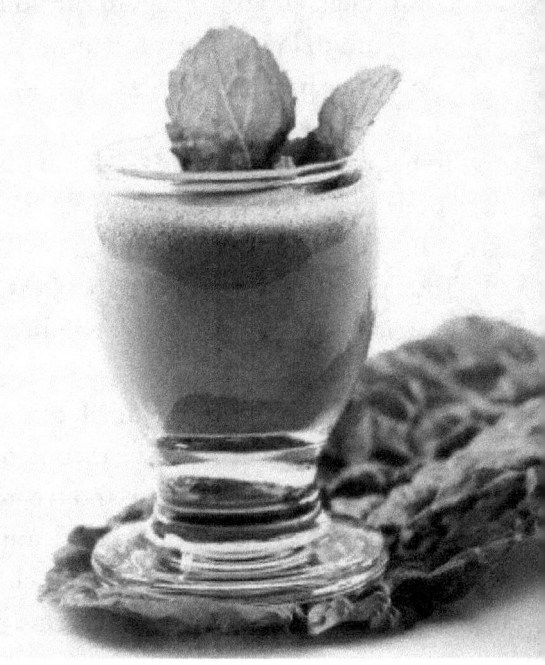

*Kale has 10 key micronutrients - low in calories, high in fiber, vitamins, and antioxidants. Coconut water is sugar, low in calories, potassium, electrolytes, minimal fat. Kale helps to support your detox cleanse and energy.

Serving Size 1 |

Ingredients:

Squeeze of lemon juice

1 cup unsweetened coconut water

¼ cup cucumber, peeled and seeded

1 cup kale leaf chunks (stems and white rib removed)

2 medium sticks of celery, chopped

¼ cup chopped flat leaf parsley

¼ cup chopped fresh mint.

¼ tsp ground or finely grated ginger

Total Carbohydrates for Recipe: 15-20 grams (mainly from coconut water, cucumber, kale, celery, and small amounts from parsley, mint, and ginger). Sugar: Negligible Protein: 3-5 grams (mainly from kale, celery, parsley)

Fat: Negligible Fiber: 2-4 grams (mainly from kale and celery). Total Calories: Approx 70-110 calories (mainly from coconut water)

Directions:

1. Place liquids into a blender, then all other ingredients and blend well. Hey presto, a detox wonder full of fiber and energy.

Notes - I use flat leaf Italian parsley but the curly variety is good too. Use what you have on hand. Interchange leafy greens to go with kale if preferred. Try Wheatgrass in place of kale. Add stevia for sweetness. Ginger is known for its anti-inflammatory properties.

Fresh Shrimp Seafood Salad

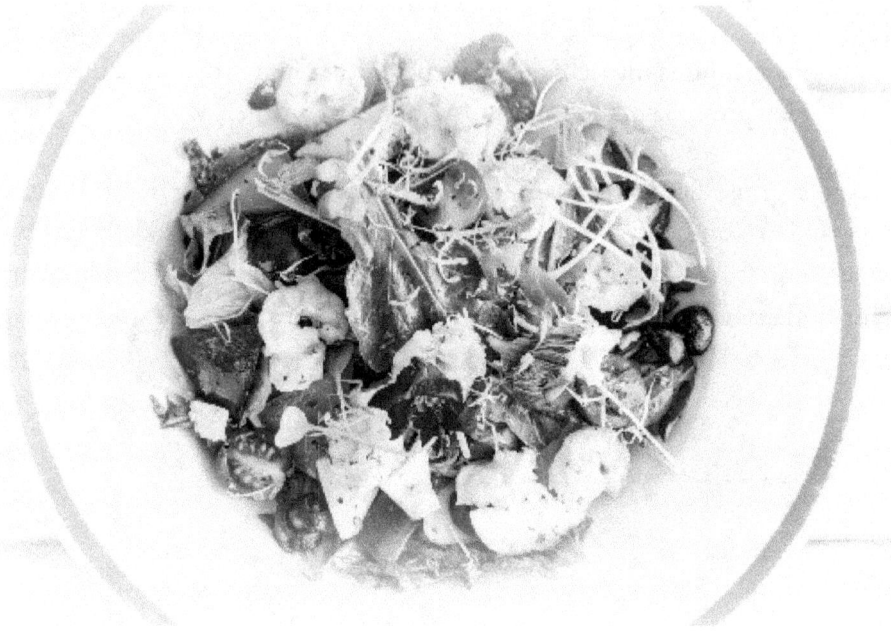

Serving size 1 |

Ingredients:

140g (3/4 cup) fresh shrimp, prawn, tuna or crab. canned or cooked and peeled

Mixed greens of your choice

1 medium-sized fresh tomato, diced

Olive oil and vinegar dressing

Optional Extras:

1/2 cup **Yellow bell** pepper 4-5g carbs.

1/4 cup **black olives** 1g carbs, 3-4g fat (olive oils)

1/4 cup **sunflower/pepita seeds** 2g carbs,1g sugar, 2g fibre,15g healthy fat.

Total Carbohydrates for Recipe: Approx. 5 grams without extras and 15 grams with extras Sugars: Less than 1 gram Protein: Approx. 6-7 grams Fat: Approx. 12-14 grams Fiber: Approx. 2-3 grams Total Calories: Approx. 200-260 calories

Directions:

1. Prepare the Shrimp: Cook the fresh shrimp by boiling, grilling, or sautéing until they turn pink and opaque. Peel and devein the shrimp if necessary, then allow them to cool.

2. Prepare the Salad: Wash and thoroughly dry the mixed greens. Place the greens in a large salad bowl.

3. Assemble the Salad: Add the cooked and peeled fresh shrimp to the mixed greens.

4. Drizzle the olive oil and vinegar dressing over the salad. You can adjust the amount of dressing to your taste. Toss the salad gently to evenly coat the ingredients with the dressing.

Notes - Serve your Fresh Shrimp Salad immediately. I had harvested my own tomatoes so they were always abundant! You can garnish it with additional toppings like cucumber slices, or sunflower seeds if desired.

Black Chia Seed Water

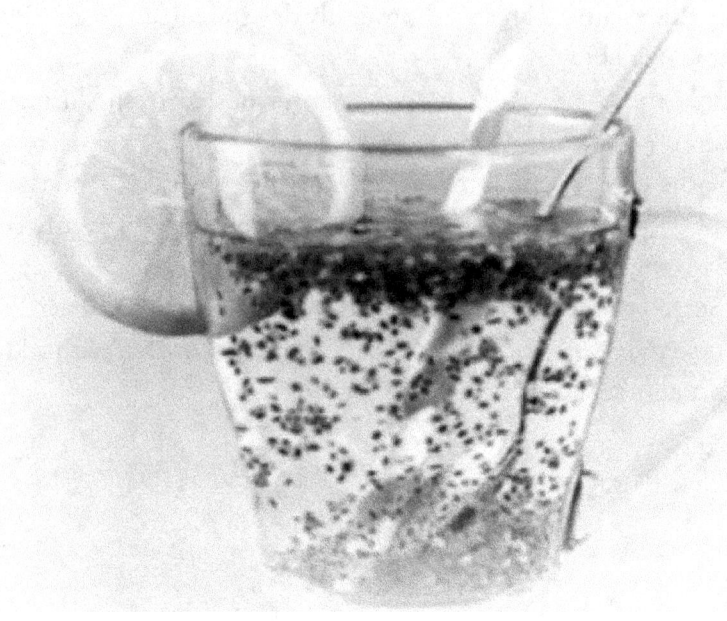

Serving size 1 | Consume half at a time, at meal times.

Ingredients:
1/2 tsp black chia seeds 1/2 glass water
squeeze of lemon (optional)
1 tsp apple cider vinegar (optional)

Directions:

Simply mix 1/2 tsp black chia seeds into 1/2 glass water. Drink half just before lunch, and the other just before dinner.

Notes - Although Chia seeds are high in protein and dietary fibre, using only 1/2 tsp in this water gives negligible readings. Chia seeds are very low in carbohydrates and calories. When mixed with water, they absorb the liquid and form a gel-like consistency. However, due to moisture absorption, monitor your digestion and adjust accordingly. Always drink plenty of liquid. They can be used to thicken dishes. Eg. add to your Greek Yoghurt or Chia Pudding.

Crumbed Cashew Chicken

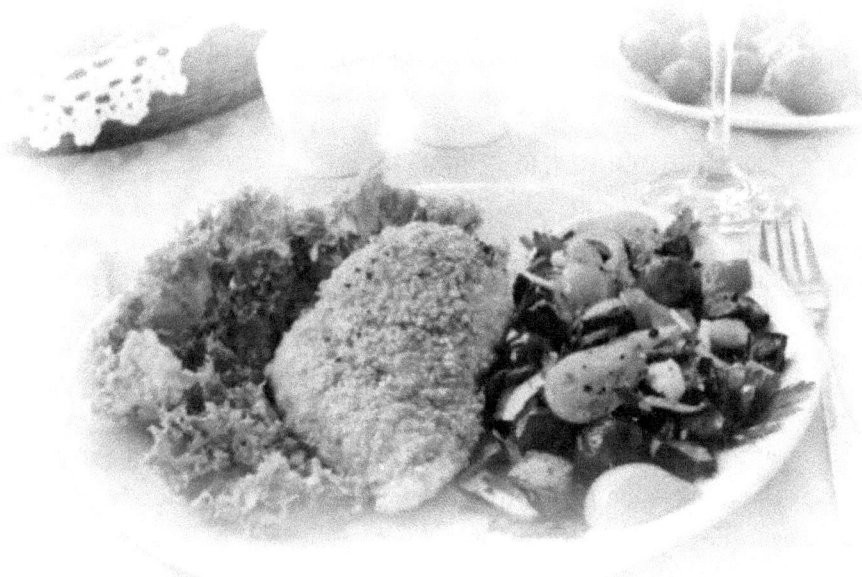

Serving size 1-2 |

Ingredients:
200g (14oz) chicken breast or skinned thigh fillets (cut into thin fillet pieces)
2 eggs, beaten
2 tsp coriander
2 tsp cumin
2 tsp ground black peppercorns
2 tsp black mustard seeds
3 Tbsp almond meal "flour" or cashew
A large pinch of salt
1 onion peeled, finely chopped (optional)
2 Tbsp Olive oil
A handful of fresh herbs - coriander, chives or parsley
*****Serve with a garden salad.**
Total Carbohydrates for Recipe: Approx. 15-18 grams Sugars: 6 grams (from almond meal or cashew meal) Protein: 75-80 grams (from chicken and

eggs) Fat: 0-45 grams (from chicken, eggs, olive oil, almond meal or cashew) Fiber: minimal Total calories: Approx. 870-900 calories

Directions:

1. In a large pie dish combine ground pepper, mustard, cumin, coriander & salt. Add almond flour. Mix well.

1. In a separate pie dish beat the eggs.

3. Dip chicken; first in egg mix. Now lift with a fork over the flour spice mix dish. generously coat chicken on both sides pressing mix in. Heat a frying pan to medium heat. 4. Transfer from dish and gently shallow fry chicken until lightly golden. In batches if necessary. -Optional side; Saute onion in another small pan for 5 minutes as a side.

Serve with a suggested large green garden salad or veg of your choice. If you want dressing, use a little olive oil and a squeeze of lemon juice, or apple cider vinegar. For a special occasion, add some lightly roasted cashew nuts on the side.

Notes: Sometimes I add sesame seeds, dried garlic or onion flakes to the almond meal mix for variety in flavors. They give a delicious nutty crunch.

Celery & Peanut Butter

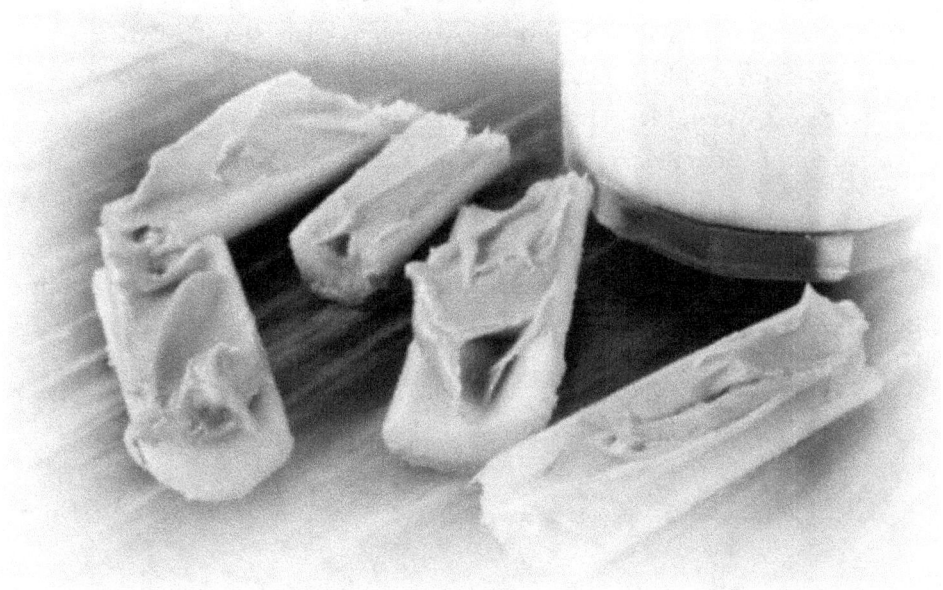

Okay, it's basic I get it... but a good old favorite when you have cravings. Tofu works in place of peanut butter if desired. Celery won't spike your insulin. The fiber content helps!

Ingredients:
2 celery stalks, chopped
1 Tbsp your favorite low sugar natural peanut butter
Total Carbohydrates for Recipe: Approx. 6-7 grams Sugars: 2-3 grams (primarily from natural peanut butter) Protein: 6-7 grams (primarily from natural peanut butter) Fat: 9-10 grams (primarily from peanut butter) Fiber: 2-3 grams (most in celery) Total Calories: 80-130 calories

Directions:
1. Wash and cut the celery into sticks.
2. Spread butter on each stalk.

Day 2

Before Breakfast: A Glass of Water Breakfast: Scrambled Egg Protein Breakfast Lunch: Baked Salmon & Asparagus with Roasted Brussels Sprouts Dinner: Homemade Beef Stew Snacks: Celery Beverages: Water, Herbal Tea or Coffee (no sweetener or milk)

Nutritional Breakdown is Per Recipe (Carbs, Sugars, Protein, Fat, Fiber and Calories.) Divide by your serving size

Net Carbs = Total Carbs – Fiber

Notes: Recipe measurements are designed for easy flexibility. Add chopped chives or garlic to the scramble eggs for some variety. Surprisingly chili works well also.

Protein Breakfast

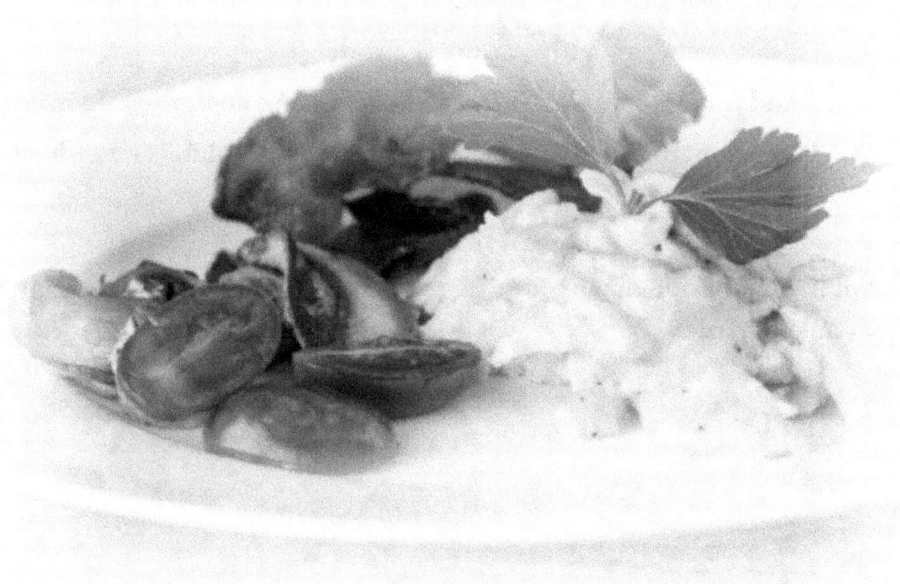

Another favourite "go to" breakfast. No toast!
Serving size 1 |
Ingredients:
2 tsps olive oil
2 eggs, beaten together in a glass
Optional: add 1 Tbsp heavy cream (negligible carbs/sugar)
1 large rasher of bacon, halved
1 small tomato, sliced
4 button mushrooms, halved black pepper to taste
Total Carbohydrates for Recipe: Approx. 4-5 grams (primarily from the tomato and mushrooms) Sugars: 2-4 grams (tomato) Protein: 15- 20 grams Fat: 25-30 grams Fiber: 1-2 grams (mushrooms) Total Calories: Approx. 350 - 410 calories (varies based on the specific preparation and size of ingredients)
Directions:

1. Over a medium heat, fry bacon until crispy in a pan with a little olive oil.
2. Add mushrooms for the last minute or so. Remove from the pan and set aside.
3. Add remainder of oil. Place the eggs in and cook for 1 - 2 mins.
4. Place tomato, egg, bacon and mushroom on a plate. Garnish with parsley if desired

Notes: Sunny side up anyone? Egg yolks retain more of their vitamins if not cooked hard.

Baked Salmon & Asparagus

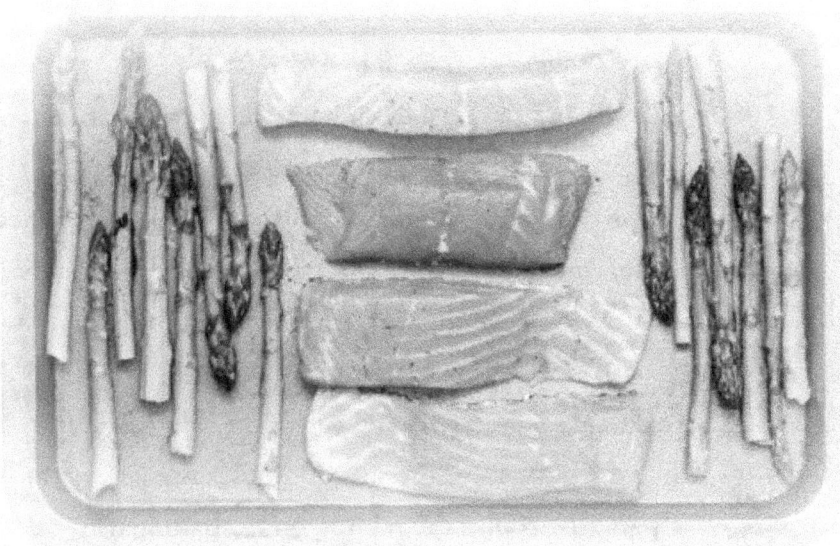

The benefits of salmon include being a rich source of omega-3 fatty acids, which support heart health, reduce inflammation, and provide essential nutrients for brain and overall well-being.

Serving size 1-2 |

Ingredients:

300 gms/ 1 1/4 cups of salmon fillet

1 cup of fresh asparagus spears

2 Tbsp of avocado oil

2 cloves of garlic, minced optional

1 lemon, thinly sliced

Optional: 1 tsp of dried thyme optional (or fresh thyme sprigs, or rosemary)

Salt and pepper, or lemon pepper to taste

Total Carbohydrates for Recipe: 7-10 grams Sugars: Approx. 2-4 grams Protein: Approx. 40-45 grams Fat: Approx. 25-30 grams Fiber: Approx. 3-4 grams Total Calories: Approx. 650-700 calories

Directions:

1. Preheat your oven to 375°F (190°C).
2. Place the salmon fillet on a baking tray lined with parchment paper or lightly greased.
3. Drizzle the avocado oil over the salmon and rub it with minced garlic. Season the salmon with salt, pepper, and dried thyme. If using fresh thyme, tuck the sprigs under the salmon for added flavor.
4. Arrange the lemon slices on top of the salmon fillet.
5. Wash and trim the woody ends of the asparagus. Lay the asparagus around the salmon on the baking tray.
6. Drizzle a little oil over the asparagus and season with salt and pepper.
7. Cover the baking tray with foil and bake in the preheated oven for about 12-15 minutes.
8. Remove the foil and continue baking for an additional 10-12 minutes or until the salmon is cooked through and flakes easily with a fork. The asparagus should be tender but still crisp.
9. Serve the baked salmon and asparagus hot, with the following brussel sprouts recipe on the side.

Notes: When my potted rosemary is growing well, I add that as my herb placing underneath and on top, but pick your favourite. Garlic works well with this recipe also.

Roasted Brussels Sprouts

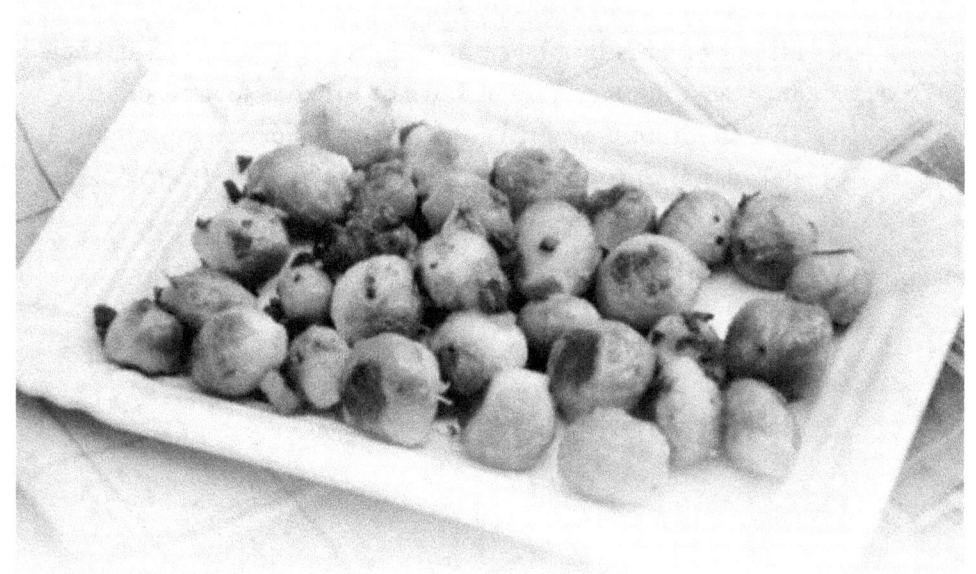

Brussels sprouts are low in calories and rich in vitamins, especially vitamin K and vitamin C. They provide fiber, which supports digestion, and are packed with antioxidants that may reduce inflammation and promote heart health.

Serving size 1-2 | Refrigerate leftovers.

Ingredients:

2 cups Brussels sprouts

1/2 onion, chopped

3 garlic cloves, finely chopped

1 Tbsp olive oil

Salt to taste

Total Carbohydrates for Recipe: Approx. 20-25 grams Sugars: 5-7 grams (from Brussels sprout and onions) Protein: 5-7 grams Fat: 7-9 grams (primarily from olive oil) Fiber: 7-9 grams (primarily from Brussels sprouts) Total Calories: Approx. 235-270 calories

Directions:

Preheat the oven to 375°F (190°C).

Toss all ingredients in a large mixing bowl. Line a baking sheet with parchment paper and place a single layer of Brussels sprouts on it.

Roast for 30 minutes or until golden brown. Serve with salmon.

Notes: Brussels Sprouts really do take better baked not steamed. Try them, but don't overcook.

Homemade Beef Stew

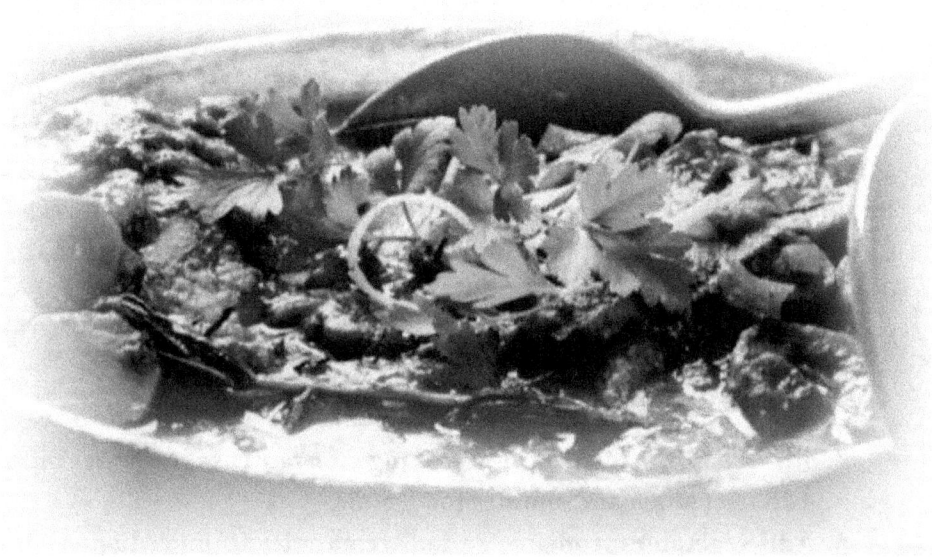

Beef is a nutrient-dense protein source rich in essential nutrients like iron, zinc, and B vitamins. It supports muscle growth, provides iron for energy, and is touted to aid in overall health when consumed as part of a balanced diet. Gives satiety and hearty satisfaction.

Serving size 4-6 | Refrigerate leftovers or freeze
Ingredients:
1 lb (450g) cubed beef stew meat
1 Tbsp of avocado or olive oil
1 onion, chopped
2 carrots, cut into pieces
1 cup homemade beef stock (or store bought or water)
1 large bell pepper, cubed
1 cups cauliflower, cut into pieces
4 mushrooms

1 800g large can tomatoes undrained (or Passata)
1 cup cabbage chopped
1/2 tsp dried rosemary (or fresh sprig)
1/2 tsp dried parsley
1 tsp ground paprika
Salt and ground black pepper to taste

Total Carbohydrates for Recipe: Approx. 15-20 grams Sugars: Approx. 8-10 grams (primarily from the vegetables and tomatoes) Protein: 25-30 grams (varies based on serving size) Fat: 10-15 grams (varies based on serving size) Fiber: 4-6 grams (primarily from veg and tomatoes) Total Calories: Approx. 1,290 or 250-300 calories per serving (varies based on serving size)

Directions:
1. Brown beef in a large heavy based pot, remove and set aside.
2. Sauté onions and carrots until golden. Return beef to the pot.
3. Stir in paprika for 1 minute stirring constantly so it doesn't burn.
4. Add beef stock and simmer for 1 hour.
5. Add vegetables, tomato, and all remainder of ingredients. Simmer for 60-80 minutes, or until tender. Adjust seasoning.

Notes: May use crockpot. Versatile stew with homemade stock, flexible ingredients, chili, homemade stock. Good for using up veg. Slow cook for tenderness & flavour. Big recipe, you'll get leftovers to freeze.

Natural Nut Mix

Eat in moderation | Serving size 2-3

Up to 1/4 cup of any mix of natural raw nuts for a snack only when you feel hungry and calories are low.

Almonds, Brazil Nuts, Walnuts, Cashews, Sunflower Seeds, Pepita Seeds.

Add salt, chili flakes, dried or mixed herbs to your preference.

Total Carbohydrates for recipe: Approx 6-8 grams Sugars: 1-2 grams (primarily from the natural sugars in the nuts and seeds) Protein: 7-9 grams Fat: 17-19 grams (primarily from the nuts and seeds) Fiber: 3-4 grams (primarily from the nuts and seeds) Total Calories: Approx. 200-280 calories

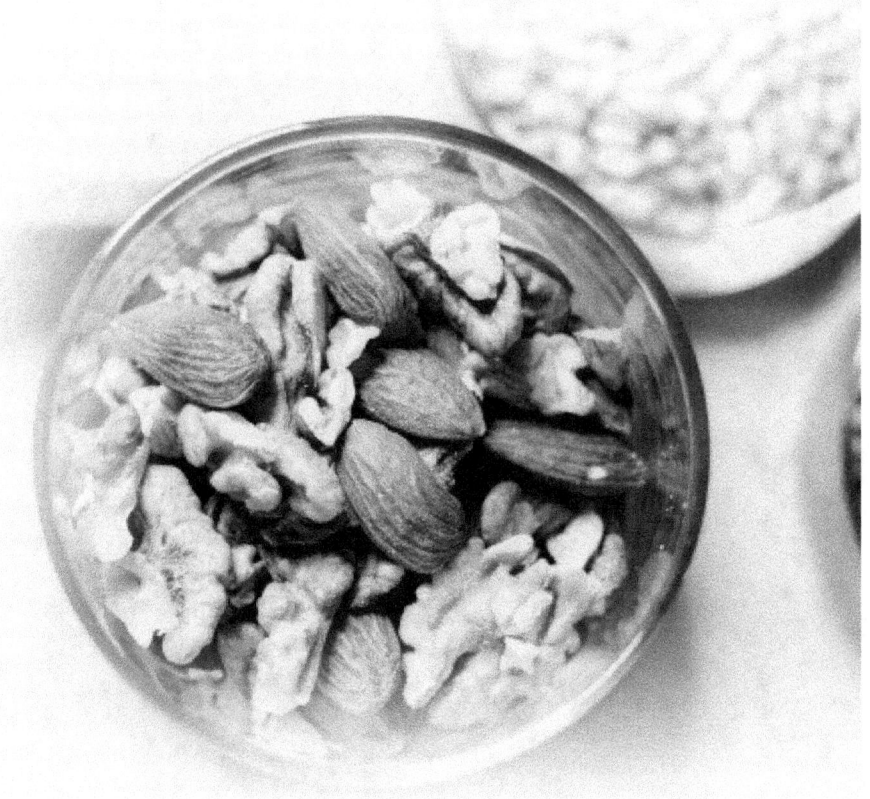

Notes: Choose nut varieties you like. Nutritious and tasty.

Day 3

Before Breakfast: A Glass of Water
Breakfast: Green Breakfast Smoothie with Bacon and Egg Chili Muffin
Lunch: Tuna Prawn & Avo Egg Salad with Low Carb Dressing
Dinner: Protein Cauli Rice Stir Fry and Spiced Choc Chia Pudding
Snacks: Celery / Chia water
Beverages: Water, Herbal Tea or Coffee (no sweetener or milk)
Nutritional Breakdown is Per Recipe (Carbs, Sugars, Protein, Fat, Fiber and Calories.) Divide by your serving size
Net Carbs = Total Carbs – Fiber

Green Breakfast Smoothie

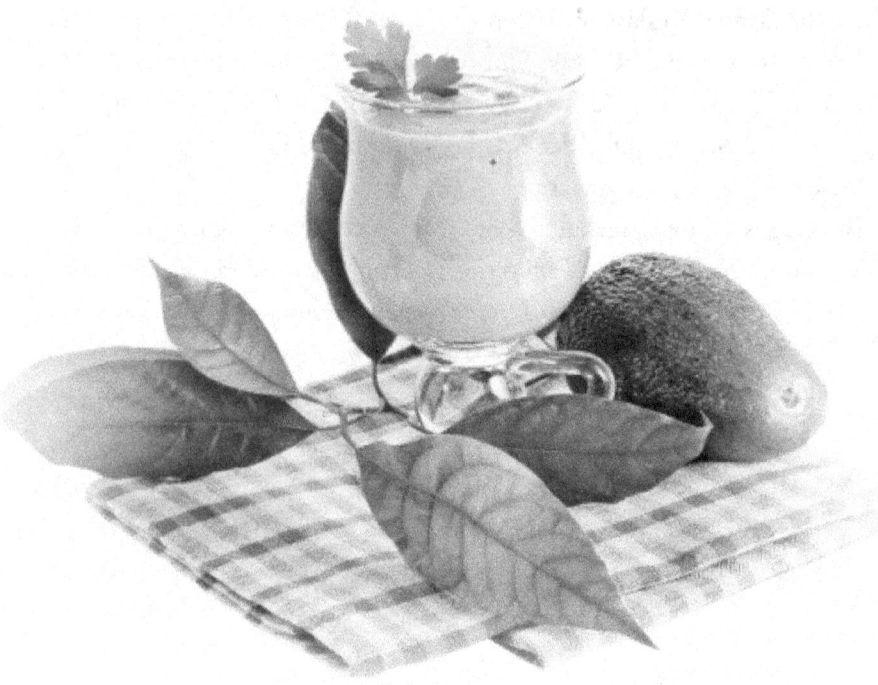

This smoothie offers hydration, vitamins, healthy fats, and fiber for skin health, energy, and digestion support.

Serving size 1 |

Ingredients:
1 Cup unsweetened coconut water
1/2 cucumber, peeled, seeded and chopped
1/2 avocado, seeded and peeled
1 - 2 sticks of celery
1\4 tsp stevia optional

Total Carbohydrates for Recipe: 15-18 grams (mainly the cucumber and avo) Total Sugars: 3-5 grams (natural sugars) Protein: 2-3 grams (mainly from avocado, some celery) Total Fat: 12-15 grams (mainly from the avocado) Fiber: 6-8 grams (mainly from cucumber and avocado) Calories: Approx. 190-230 calories

Directions:
1. Prepare ingredients then add cold coconut water to the blender first.
2. Place all other ingredients in and whiz it up till smooth.

Notes: Experiment with leafy greens and avo. The other half can be used for the dinner recipe. Be sure this avocado is very ripe for a smooth mixture. You can have this recipe with lunch also.

Bacon & Egg Chili Muffin

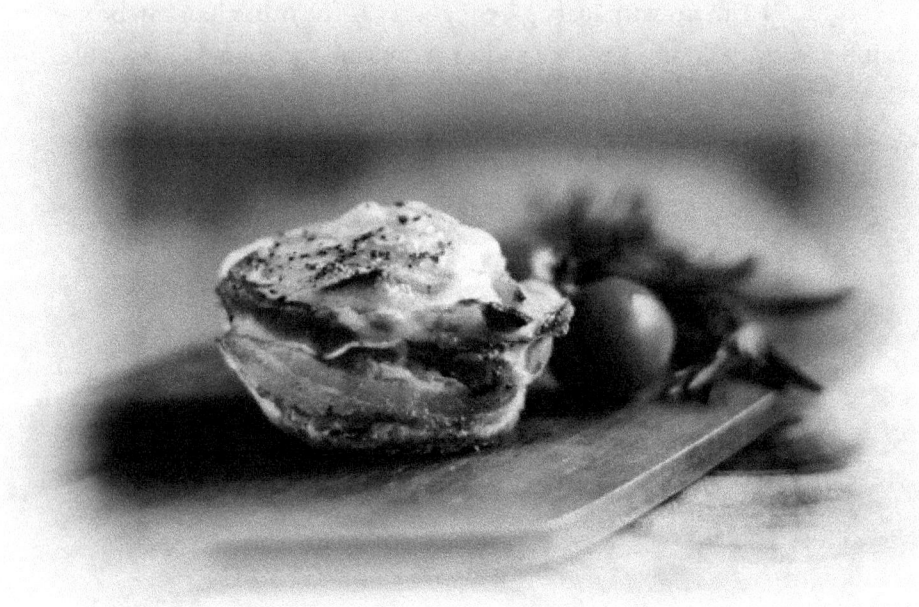

Serving size 2-4 | Refrigerate leftovers

Ingredients:
Olive oil cooking spray
4 slices bacon
4 large eggs
1 tsp ground black pepper
1/4 cup sliced green onions / chives (optional)
1/4 cup diced med-hot chili peppers (optional)
1/4 cup almond meal
1/2 cup crumbled low carb tofu (firm tofu works well)
1/4 cup heavy cream
Total Carbohydrates for Recipe: Approx. 6-8 grams Sugar: 2 grams

Protein: 12 grams Fat: 16 grams Fiber: 2 grams Calories: Approx. 750 - 810 calories

Directions:

1. Preheat the oven to 375 degrees F (190 degrees C). Grease a 6 cup muffin tin with cooking spray.
2. Arrange bacon on a microwave-safe plate. Microwave on high for 75 seconds.
3. Line each muffin cup with one bacon slice going around the edges of the cup.
4. In a bowl, mix eggs, heavy cream, salt, and pepper together. Add any greens or chili. Stir in crumbled tofu and almond meal.
5. Spoon the egg mixture into the muffin cups.
6. Bake until the top looks done, about 15 minutes.

Serve with cherry tomatoes or salad and chia water.

Notes: I adjust this recipe depending on my mood. Sometimes just eggs and bacon. Try different greens and chili, even chili paste. Try mozzarella on top. Add a pinch of onion flakes, or herbs on top for crunch. Create your own for any meal of the day!

The almond meal gives a little crust at base and provides some extra protein. Microwave and eat leftovers the next day or freeze.

Tuna Prawn & Avo Egg Salad

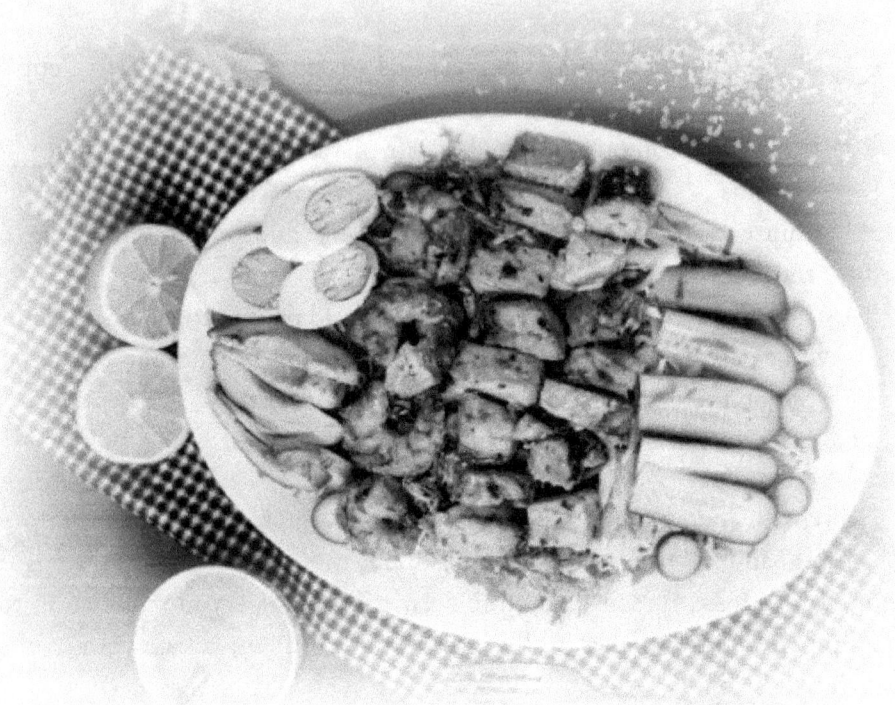

Combining tuna and prawns for high protein, low-carb, and omega-3-rich health benefits, supporting heart health and muscle development. Dress up with a simple drizzle of olive oil or make up your own low carb recipe.

Serving size 1-2 | Refrigerate leftovers

Ingredients:

1 Medium can (185g) or fresh, or drained canned tuna chunks in oil (salmon, or sardines are also good. Try to buy pole or line caught not farmed; their diet is natural not grain fed)

150 gms of cooked prawn or shrimp

Optional 1 hard boiled egg, halved.

1/2 avocado, sliced

1-2 Tbsp mix of: sesame seed oil and Dijon mustard.

1-2 Tbsp of cucumber chopped

1-2 Tbsp of chopped red onion (optional)

Salt, pepper to taste
A squeeze of lemon juice (optional)
Fresh herbs and sesame seeds for garnish (optional)
Total Carbohydrates for Recipe: Approx. 9-12 grams Sugars: 1-2 grams (primarily from vegetables) Protein: 30-35 grams Fat: 20-25 grams (may vary based on the amount of sesame seed oil and other ingredients used) Total Calories: Approx. 650-710 calories

Directions:

1. In a large salad bowl, gently combine drained tuna, cooked prawns / shrimp, and hard-boiled egg halves.

2. Add the sliced avocado to the bowl. The avocado's creamy texture complements the seafood.

3. In a separate small bowl, whisk together the sesame seed oil and Dijon mustard. Adjust the quantities to your taste. I use half and half.

4. Pour the sesame seed oil and Dijon mustard mixture over the salad ingredients.

5. Add the remaining cucumber and red onion to the salad for freshness and crunch.

Arrange creatively on the plate as you choose.

Drizzle with Low Carb Salad Dressing next.

Notes: Another super flexible lunch recipe. This is so packed full of energy and goodness I often use as a dinner recipe too. Change it up by removing prawns and adding nuts and seeds.

Low Carb Salad Dressing

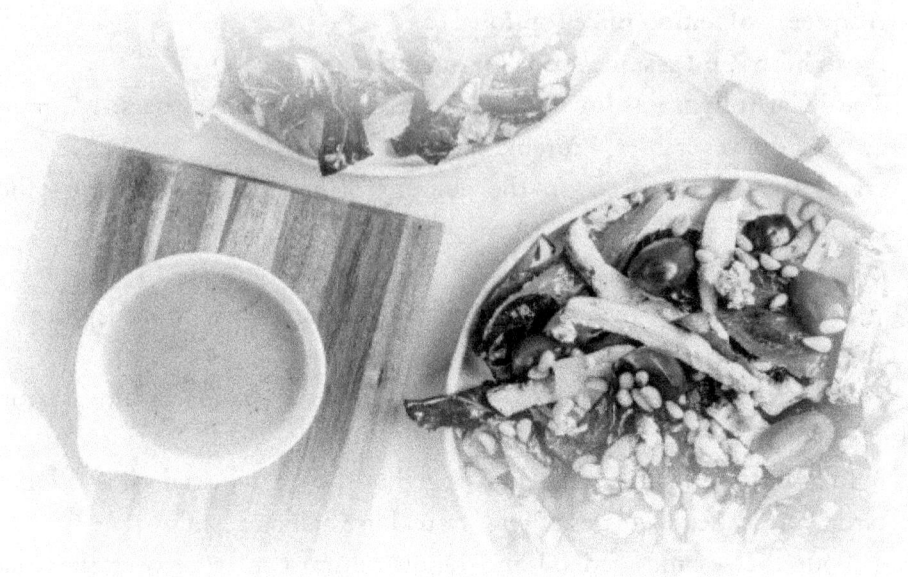

Use extra virgin olive oil as a base in your dressings.

Olive oil is rich in heart healthy monounsaturated fats and antioxidants. It can help absorption of fat-soluble nutrients in salads, such as vitamins A, D, E, and K.

Serving size 4-6 |

Ingredients:
2 Tbsp olive oil
1 Tbsp apple cider vinegar (make sure it's sugar-free)
1/2 tsp Dijon mustard (check for added sugars)
1 small clove of garlic, minced (optional)
pinch of herbs of your choice (optional)

Total Carbohydrates for Recipe: Very low, primarily from the apple cider vinegar). Sugars: Minimal, depending on the apple cider vinegar and Dijon mustard. Protein: Negligible. Fat: Mainly from olive oil; about 28 grams in total.

Fiber: Negligible. Calories: Approx. 240-250 for the whole recipe.
Directions:

1. In a small bowl, whisk together the olive oil, apple cider vinegar, and Dijon mustard. The mustard helps with emulsification and adds flavor.
2. Add the minced garlic if you like a garlicky flavor. You can adjust the amount as desired.
3. Season with salt if you prefer, pepper and herbs of choice.
4. Whisk all the ingredients together until well combined.
5. Taste and adjust the seasoning. Add a little more vinegar or oil to adjust the consistency.

Notes: Use this on any salad. Cover and place leftovers in the fridge. Try using about 1 Tbsp of mashed avocado in place of the mustard. I do this when a meal includes an avo salad.

NOTES

Protein Cauli Rice Stir Fry

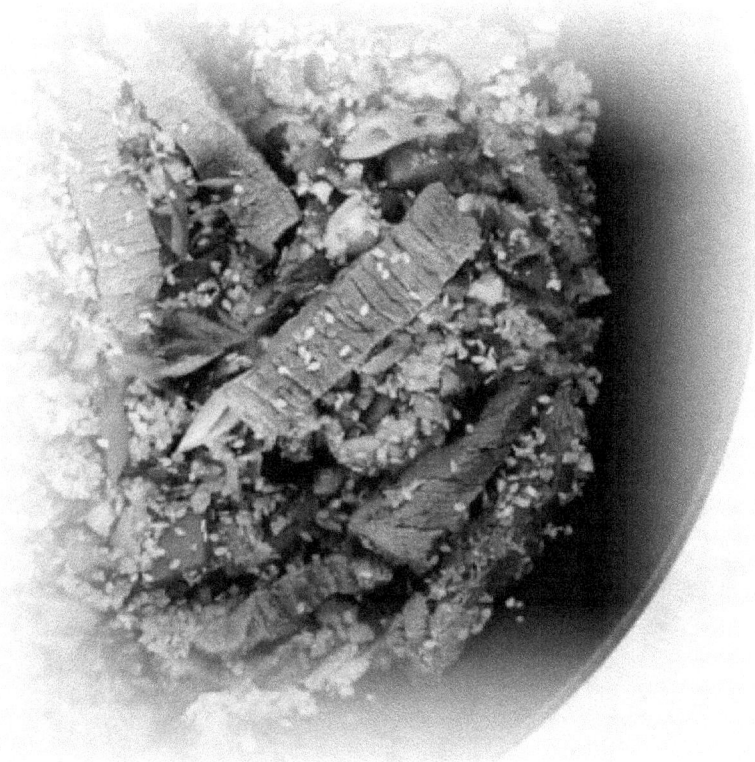

Protein and vitamin rich for sustained energy.

Serving size 4-6 | Refrigerate leftovers or freeze

Ingredients:

1 head of cauliflower (to make cauliflower rice)

2 cups finely sliced assorted stir-fry vegetables (e.g., broccoli, spring onions, sweet potato or bell peppers)

400 gms protein, sliced (beef, pork, chicken, shrimp, etc.)

1 tsp sesame oil

2 tsp sesame seeds (optional)

1 tsp coconut oil

1 Tbsp low carb soy sauce or coconut aminos

Fresh ginger to taste (I grate about 1 tsp fresh ginger)

3 cloves of garlic

Total Carbohydrates for Recipe: Approx. 23-28 grams Sugars: 5-7 grams (primarily from vegetables) Protein: 30-35 grams (varies based on the type of protein used) Fat: 10-15 grams (may vary based on the type and amount of oil used) Fiber: 7-10 grams Total Calories: Approx. 730-820 calories

Directions:

1. Grate or process the cauliflower into rice-like pieces.
2. On a high heat, use a fry pan or wok with a little oil and stir-fry your choice of protein with garlic, ginger, adding a small amount of soy sauce or coconut aminos. Add a splash of water if required.
3. Remove from wok and place aside on a warmed large serving dish.
4. Quickly stir fry the remaining vegetables with oil for a few minutes.
5. Add the cauliflower rice to stir-fry vegetables and protein back into wok to gently combine. Cook for 1-2 minutes until everything is tender.

Finish with a drizzle of sesame oil and garnish with scallions or chopped spring onions if preferred.

Notes: Sometimes I swap the veggies around. Use what you have in the fridge. Ginger and garlic may be doubled if you prefer.

Spiced Choc Chia Pudding

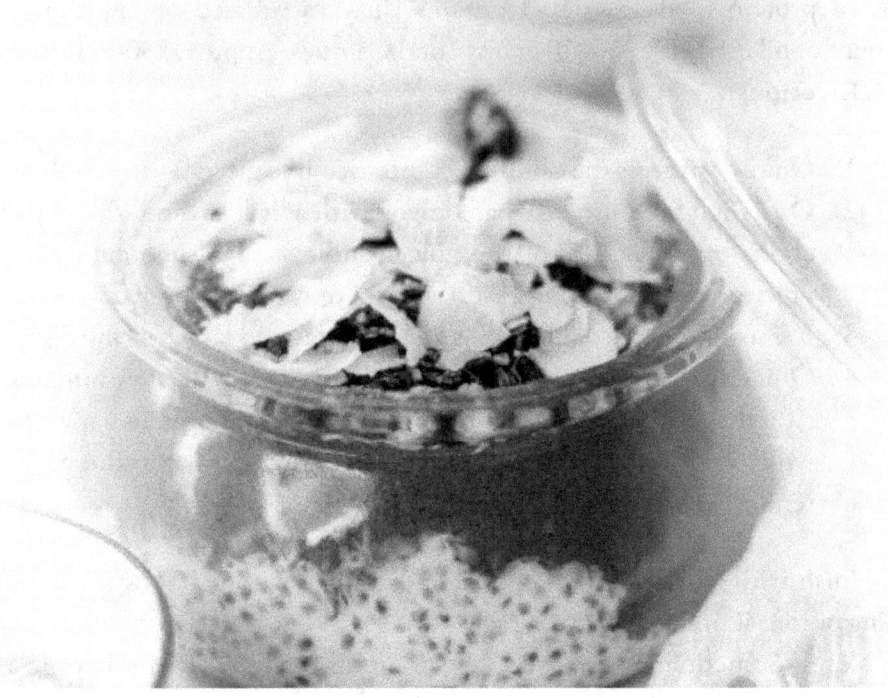

Black chia seeds are rich in fiber, omega-3 fatty acids, antioxidants, and may support heart health, digestion and weight management.

Serving size 4 | Keep sealed in the fridge, use up in 4 days or freeze into smaller pudding cups.

Ingredients:
4 Tbsp whole black chia seeds
1/4 cup heavy cream
1 cup water (or unsweetened coconut milk)
1 Tbsp raw cacao powder or Dutch cocoa powder
2 tsp monk fruit powder
5 drops Stevia extract (optional)
1 tsp raw cacao nibs (or raw crushed nuts)
A large pinch of coconut flakes to garnish
Total Carbohydrates for Recipe: Approx. 25 grams Sugars: 2-4 grams (natural sugars and sweeteners) Protein: 5-8 grams Fat: 30-35 grams Fiber:

10-15 grams (from chia, cocoa) Total Calories: Approx. 550-600 calories for recipe

Directions:

1. In a mixing bowl, combine the chia seeds, heavy cream, water (or almond milk), and raw cacao powder (or cocoa powder). Whisk well to ensure the cocoa is evenly distributed and chia seeds separated.

2. Add the monk fruit powder and Stevia extract to the mixture. Adjust the sweetness and cocoa to your taste.

3. Transfer the mixture into a serving glass or jar.

4. Sprinkle the raw cocoa nibs (or raw nuts) on top of the pudding for added texture and flavor. Lastly add the coconut flakes on top to garnish.

Refrigerate the pudding for at least 2 hours, or overnight, to allow the chia seeds to absorb the liquid and create a pudding-like texture. Serve chilled.

(OR method 2: Mix separately - cacao, stevia and 1 tsp water. Blend through the top of the pudding after step 3.)

Notes: Refrigerate and enjoy sweets over the next few days. I like to use coconut milk. The cacao nibs and coconut flakes go soft overnight, simply delicious!

Day 4

Before Breakfast: A Glass of Water

Breakfast: Pan Fried Omelet & Chia Avocado Dip

Lunch: Chili Pork Patties with Tomato and Basil

Snacks: A Few Raw Nuts or Celery

Dinner: BBQ Jalapeño Mint Lamb with Cauliflower Mash

Snacks: A Few Raw Nuts

Beverages: Water, or Chia Water, Herbal Tea or Coffee (no sweetener or milk)

Nutritional Breakdown is Per Recipe (Carbs, Sugars, Protein, Fat, Fiber and Calories.) Divide by your serving size

Net Carbs = Total Carbs − Fiber

Notes: Use up leftover Chia Pudding from yesterday when hungry at breakfast or lunch time. If not, use it at lunch time

Pan Fried Omelette

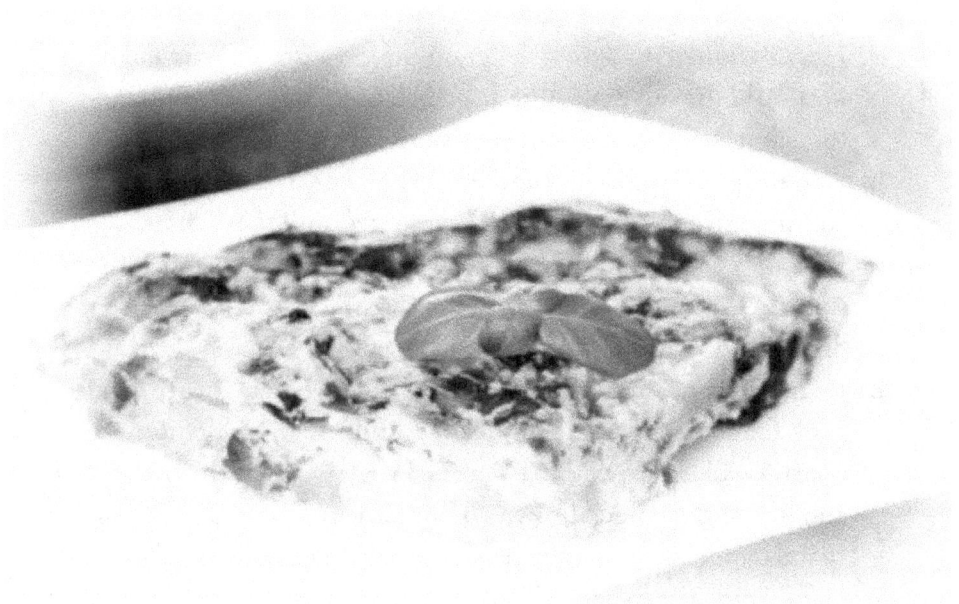

Serving Size 2 | Refrigerate or freeze leftovers
  Ingredients:
  4 large eggs
  1 Tbsp heavy/whole cream
  1/2 cup diced bell peppers (any color you prefer)
  1/2 cup diced onions (red or white)
  1/2 cup diced spinach or any leafy greens
  Salt and pepper to taste
  1/2 tsp flaked chili (optional)
  1/2 tsp mixed dried herbs (optional)
  2 tsp olive oil or olive oil cooking spray
  Total Carbohydrates for Recipe: Approx. 16-20 grams (mostly from vegetables). Sugars: 6-8 grams (natural sugars from vegetables). Protein: 20-24 grams. Fat: 32-36 grams Fiber: 3-5 grams
  Calories: 450-650 calories for the entire frittata.
  Directions:

1. In a mixing bowl, whisk eggs and cream until well combined. Season with salt and pepper. Add dried herbs and chili flakes if using. Set this mixture aside.

1. Heat a 10-inch non-stick skillet on the gas stovetop over medium heat. Add the olive oil. Add diced bell peppers and onions and sauté for about 3-5 minutes until they start to soften.
2. Add the diced spinach (or other leafy greens) to the skillet and continue to cook for another 1-2 minutes until they wilt.
3. Pour the egg and cream mixture over the sautéed vegetables in the skillet. Gently stir the mixture to ensure the vegetables are evenly distributed.
4. Reduce the heat to low and cover with a lid. Allow the frittata to cook for about 5 minutes or until it is fully set in the center. Occasionally lift the lid to check its progress. Once the frittata is set and has a light golden brown color on the bottom, carefully slide a spatula under it to make sure it's not sticking to the pan.
5. Gently flip over to cook the other side for an extra 5 minutes, or until it's set. Once cooked, slide it onto a serving plate.

Slice the frittata into wedges and serve. You can garnish with additional grated Parmesan cheese, fresh herbs, or a dollop of sour cream, if desired.

Notes: Don't overcook or this egg recipe becomes rubbery. I also use leftover vegetables, whatever is growing in my VeggiePod. Chives, Thyme, Swiss chard, broccolini and silverbeet are all good in this recipe. Try the chili in it for a change! Always remove tough stem spines as they will be chewy and undercooked... unless you have Samuri fine knife skills!!

It also makes a fabulous brunch with protein and a side sala

Chia Avocado Dip

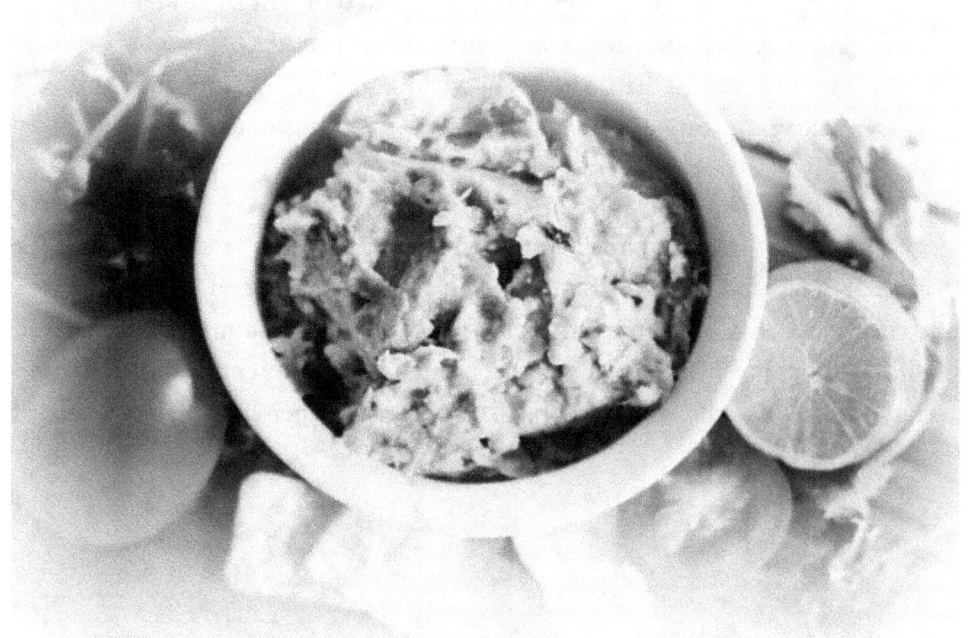

Avocados are full of healthy fats. The chia seeds will help you feel full until lunch time.

Serving size 2-3 | Keep cool in the fridge. Use up in 2 days
Ingredients:
2 ripe avocados
2 tomatoes (optional)
2 garlic cloves, minced
½ cup fresh coriander or cilantro, finely chopped
1 Tbsp lime or lemon juice
pinch of chia seeds (optional)
1/2 chopped red onion (optional)
salt and pepper to taste
Total Carbohydrates for Recipe: Approx. 35-40 grams
Sugars: 4-6 grams Protein: 5-8 grams Fat: 20-25 grams Fiber: 15-20 grams Total Calories: Approx. 500-550 calories
Directions:

1. Make sure the avocados are ripe. Peel them, cut in halves and place the pulps in a bowl.
2. Blanch tomatoes if using - Bring water to boil, put the tomatoes in the water for a minute, take them out and peel.
3. Put all the ingredients in the bowl and mash with a fork to create guacamole dip.
4. Season as desired.

Notes: Another versatile favourite is the avocado. Use sliced, pureed or mashed - in salads, dips, with eggs and meals in general. Avocado is a nutrient-dense fruit known for its heart-healthy monounsaturated fats, rich in fiber, vitamins, and minerals. It supports weight management, skin health, and is touted to reduce the risk of heart disease due to its beneficial fat profile and other nutrients.

Chili Pork Protein Patties

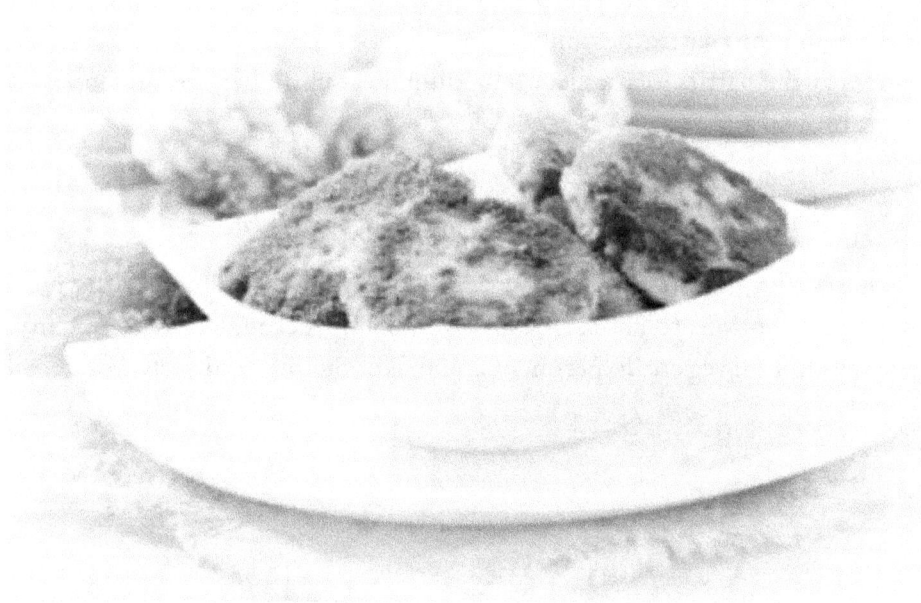

Use any protein you desire such as chicken, beef, lamb, firm fish etc
Serving size 4-6 | Refrigerate or freeze leftovers.

Ingredients:
1lb (450 g) lean pork, ground
1 tsp sage
1 tsp salt
1 tsp paprika powder
1/2 tsp fresh black pepper or chili flakes, ground
1/2 cup almond meal for coating
Total Carbohydrates for Recipe: Approx. 12-14 grams
Sugars: Negligible Protein: 87-92 grams Fat: 66-76 grams Fiber: 6 grams Calories: Approx. 960-1160 calories

Directions:

1. In a small bowl mix all spices together.
2. Add this mixture to the ground pork. Blend well.
3. Form into flat patties and dip into almond meal.
4. Fry the patties in a skillet on medium heat until they are golden brown.
5. Serve with Tomato and Basil Salad next.
6. Add some finely diced kale or spinach for extra goodness.

Notes: Who doesn't like a tasty pattie? Yet another flexible healthy meal with so many options to choose from. Pork, beef, chicken, lamb, Tofu, lentil, kale, spicy chili, all veg etc. Experiment and make your own uniquely wonderful creation!

Tomato and Basil Salad

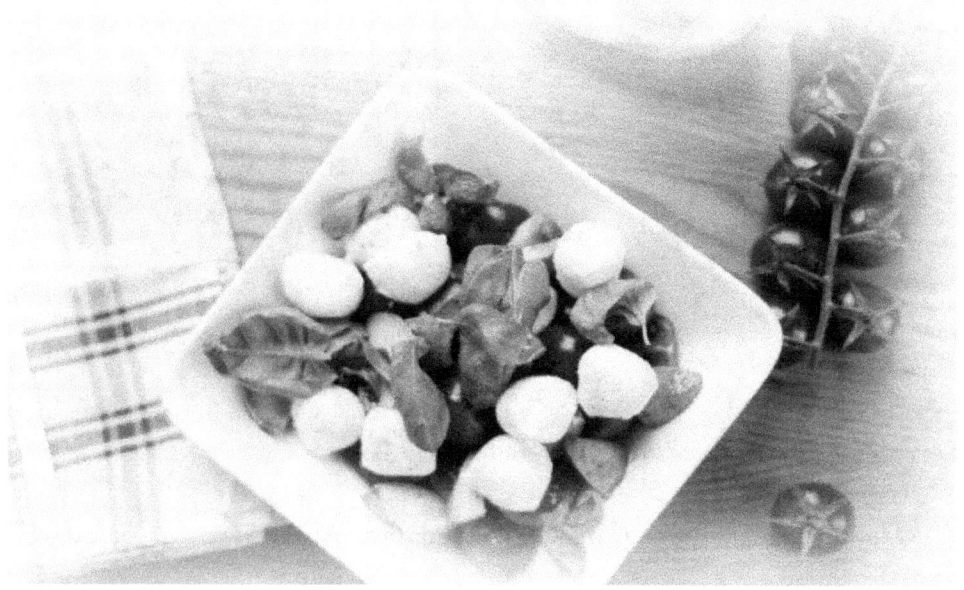

Serves 2- 4 | Refrigerate
Ingredients:
1 ripe avocado, diced
1 cup cherry tomatoes
1 cup small Mozzarella balls or Tofu
1/2 bunch of basil leaves
Olive oil and lemon juice to taste
Salt and black pepper to taste
Total Carbohydrates for Recipe: Approx. 20-24 grams

Sugars: 5-10 grams Protein: 15-20 grams Fat: 40-50 grams Fiber: 10-15 grams Total Calories: Approx. 630-690 calories

Directions:
In a small dish combine olive oil, lemon juice, salt and black pepper.

In a salad bowl mix together diced avocado, cherry tomatoes and Mozzarella balls. Pour the dressing over. Serve immediately.

BBQ Jalapeño Mint Lamb

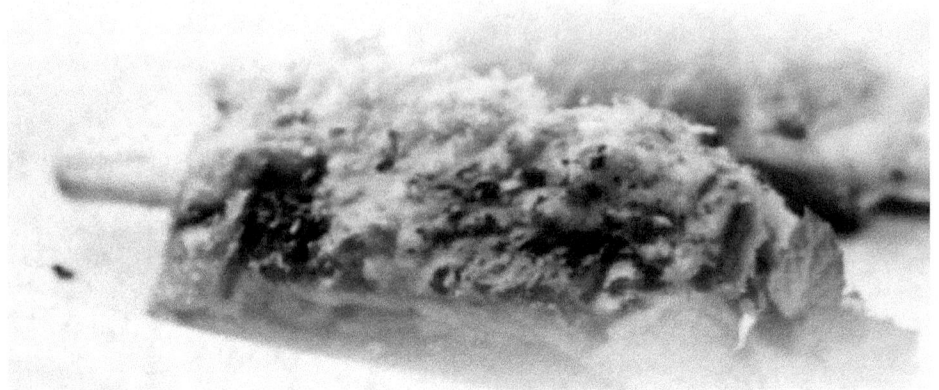

Serving size 4 | Double up sauce ingredients if desired

Ingredients:

1 lamb rack (about 1kg) may be divided into quarters if you like lamb well done

4 cloves garlic, minced or blended

2 jalapeño chilies, minced or blended

Sea salt to taste

1/4 cup low-carb mint sauce (or tomato sauce)

2-3 Tbsp olive oil

Total Carbohydrates: Around 8-10 grams

Sugars: 5-8 grams Protein: 70-80 grams Fat: 35-40 grams

Fiber: 1-2 grams Total Calories: Approx. 1,600 -1,900 calories

Directions:

1. Preheat your BBQ or grill to medium-high heat.
2. Season the lamb rack with sea salt and let it sit at room temperature for 15-30 minutes.
3. In a small bowl, mix the mint sauce, olive oil, minced garlic and jalapeño chilies ready for basting.
4. Grill the lamb for 4-6 minutes on each side to sear it and get it nicely browned (or charred) to your liking.
5. Reduce the heat to medium-low and grill.

Continually baste with sauce mix as you turn and cook for another 5-6 minutes until done as desired.

Let the lamb rest for 5-10 minutes before serving with grilled low carb vegetables and or salad.

Notes: Try using different low sugar sauces or natural homemade sauces such as olive oil, coconut oil, chopped fresh rosemary.

Cauliflower Mash

Serving size 4 | Season as you please. Refrigerate leftovers
   Ingredients:
   1 head of cauliflower
   2-3 cloves of garlic, minced (adjust to your taste)
   2-3 Tbsp butter (you can also use olive oil for a dairy-free version)
   Salt and pepper, to taste
   Optional toppings: grated Parmesan cheese, fresh herbs, or chives.
   Total Carbohydrates: Approx. 20-25 grams
   Sugars: 10-15 grams (mainly from the cauliflower) Protein: 9-15 grams Fat: 24-36 grams Fiber: 12-18 grams Total Calories: Estimated at 360-400 calories
   Directions:

1. Start by cutting the cauliflower into large florets, removing the tough stem and leaves. Rinse under cold water.In a large pot, either use a steamer, or bring water to a boil. Cook for about 10-15 minutes or until they are very tender and easily pierced with a fork.
2. Drain the cauliflower in a colander to remove excess water.
3. In a separate small pan, melt the butter (or heat the olive oil) over low heat. Add the minced garlic and sauté for a minute or two until it becomes fragrant but not browned. This will infuse the cauliflower mash with a lovely garlic flavor.
4. Place the cooked cauliflower in a food processor, blender or hand mash. Add the garlic-infused butter (or olive oil), salt, and pepper. Blend until the mixture is smooth and has the consistency of mashed potatoes.

Taste and adjust the seasoning with more salt and pepper if needed. If you'd like, top your cauliflower mash with grated Parmesan cheese, chili flakes, fresh herbs, or chives for extra flavor.

Notes: Cauliflower has less carbs and sugar than regular Mashed Potato. The flavor is very pleasant and still buttery.

Day 5

Before Breakfast: A Glass of Water
  Breakfast: Skillet Ham Steak with Asparagus & Tomato
  Lunch: Green Lentil Thai Curry
  Dinner: Grilled Steak with Rocket & Sesame Apple Cider Vinegar Coleslaw
  Snacks: Celery or Leafy greens
  Beverages: Water, Herbal Tea or Coffee, or Fresh Ginger Tea

Nutritional Breakdown is Per Recipe (Carbs, Sugars, Protein, Fat, Fiber and Calories.) Divide by your serving size
Net Carbs = Total Carbs – Fiber

Today there is a new beverage for you to try! No need to buy Ginger tea bags anymore. Homemade natural Fresh Ginger Tea tastes amazing, aids digestion and nausea, plus saves the environment and your money!

Notes: Drink more water today due to higher sodium content! Fresh Ginger Tea Recipe: With a nutmeg or fine grater, simply grate about 1/2 tsp of fresh ginger into a cup and add boiling water. Allow to steep for at least 5 minutes. Top up again with water if desired. This small amount contains a negligible amount of sugar and carbs typically less than 1g per serve. Fresh is best.

Skillet Ham Steak with Asparagus & Tomato

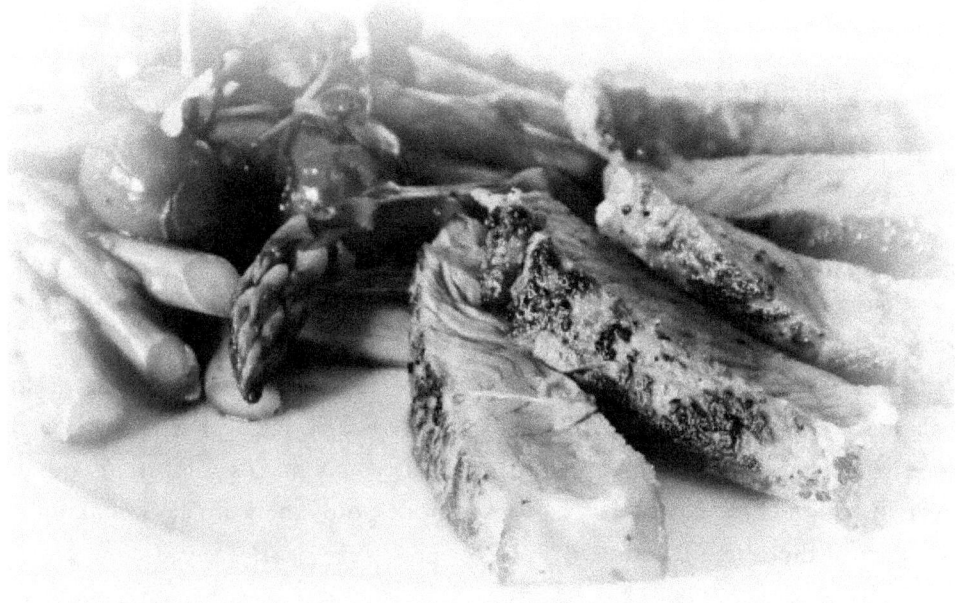

Serving Size 1-2 |
   Ingredients:
   1 thick ham steak or organic bacon strips, sliced
   6-8 asparagus spears
   3 cherry tomatoes
   3 button mushrooms (optional)
   1 Tbsp avocado OR coconut oil
   Pepper to taste
   Total Carbohydrates for Recipe: Approx. 8-10 grams Sugars: 3-7 grams Protein: 22-28 grams Fat: 10-15 grams Fiber: 4-7 grams Total Calories: Approx. 410-460 calories
   Directions:

   1. Heat a skillet over medium-high heat and add the olive or avocado

oil.
2. Season the ham steak with pepper as desired.
3. Place the ham steak in the skillet and cook for about 4-6 minutes on each side or until it's nicely browned and heated through. Remove and set aside.
4. In the same skillet, add the asparagus spears. Cook for about 3-4 minutes, or until tender and slightly charred, turning them occasionally.
5. Add the tomatoes to the skillet and cook for 1-2 minutes until it's warmed through.

Plate the ham steak, asparagus, and tomato together on a plate, and serve your delicious and nutritious breakfast.

Notes: Ham steaks and bacon contain a high sodium (salt) content so balance with asparagus, broccolini, spinach or beans. Broad beans work well too. Sometimes I add eggs and mushrooms which makes a fabulous quick brunch recipe. Avocado oil has a higher smoke point than olive oil, making it suitable for high-heat cooking.

Green Lentil Thai Curry

Lentils offer protein, fiber, vitamins, minerals, and may aid heart health, digestion, and weight management.

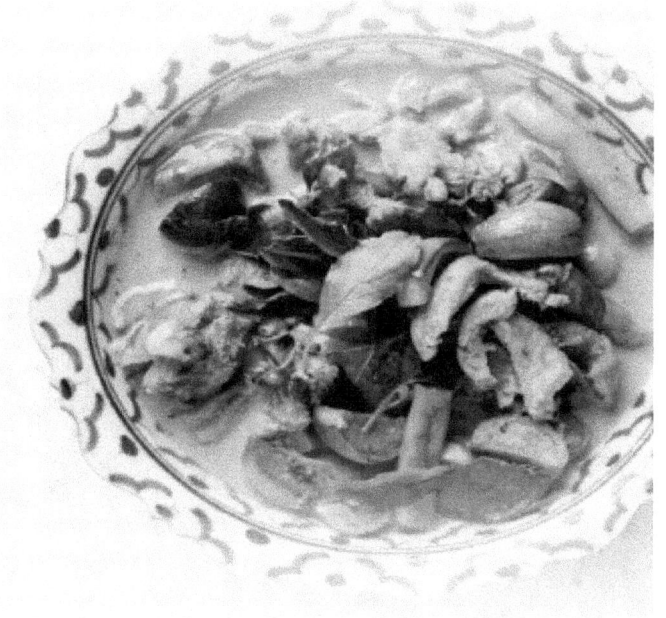

Serving size 4-6 | *Cover lentils in water & soak 1-2 hr beforehand* | Refrigerate or freeze leftovers.

Ingredients:
2 lbs (1kg) whole chicken thighs, skin off.
1/2 cup brown or green lentils (soaked in water for 1-2 hours and drained).
1 Tbsp organic coconut oil
3 cloves of garlic, roughly chopped (optional)
1-inch cube of freshly minced ginger (use a grater)
1/2 - 3/4 Tbsp Green Curry Paste (I use natural Mae Ploy)
3 fresh Kaffir lime leaves (fresh or frozen)
1 lb (500g) low-starch vegetables eg broccoli, cauliflower, zucchini, mushrooms, kale, spinach, bok choy, Swiss chard, and/or cauliflower.

1 400ml can of coconut cream (I use 100% natural Ayam).
1 cup of natural chicken stock (optional - or water; check low carb ingredients for store-bought)
1/4 tsp salt (to taste)

A small handful of chopped coriander or basil mint leaves, and/or chili for garnish (use any Asian herbs you have growing).

Serve with the Cauli Rice or extra vegetables.

Total Carbohydrates for Recipe: Approx. 70-80 grams Sugars: 4 grams Protein: 86 grams Total Fat: 56 grams Dietary Fiber: 17 grams Total Calories: 1,240-2800 calories for recipe.

Directions:

1. Slice your vegetables into large chunks, slice garlic, and grate the ginger.
2. Heat a large, heavy frying pan (with a lid) over medium-high heat.
3. Add the coconut oil and place all the chicken evenly into the pan.
4. Spread the curry paste across the chicken using a spatula or spoon, trying to coat a little on each thigh.
5. Repeat with the grated ginger, garlic, and add the salt.
6. Lay the lime leaves across the top.
7. Fry the chicken until golden on one side, about 15 minutes.
8. Turn over each chicken thigh, then pour in the stock , coconut milk, and stir in the lentils.
9. Sit all the vegetables evenly on top.
10. Simmer on low for another 20-30 minutes until done. Garnish with fresh herbs from your garden, such as basil mint, or coriander.

Notes: One of my favourite dinner recipes. A tasty BIG one pot recipe is plenty for all! I use homemade stock to enhance flavor, provide nutrients, and reduce food waste. Cooking time varies depending on the size of chicken. One of the best potted plant investments has to be my Kaffir Lime tree. The Flavor is better than store bought and the leaves are organic! I grate the ginger straight into the pan over the chicken. Too spicy hot? We've all been there... just add Greek yogurt or fresh cucumber as a side. If you want less carbs, remove lentils.

Grilled Steak with Rocket

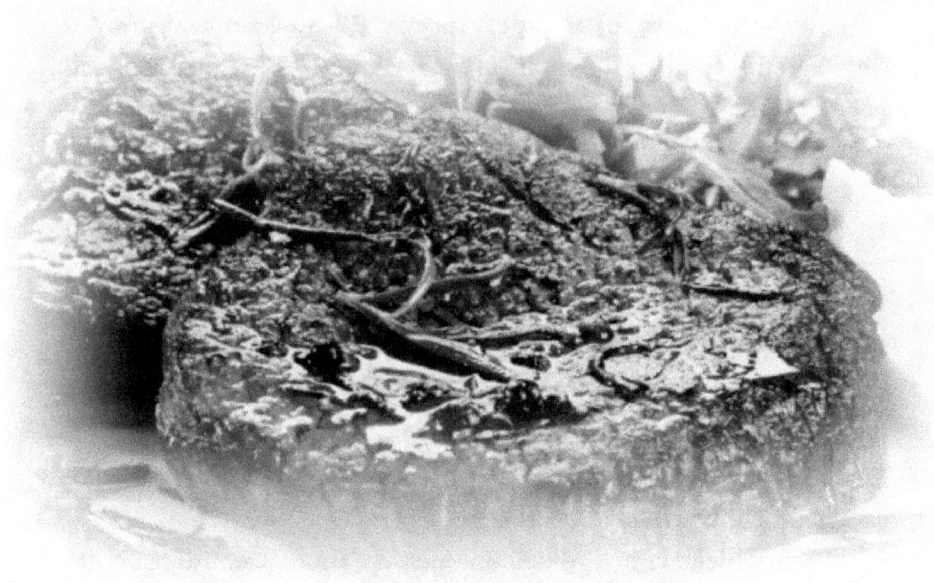

This grilled steak with rocket and pomegranate seeds is a protein-rich dish that offers iron, vitamins, minerals, antioxidants, and healthy fats.

Serving Size 1 |

Ingredients:
1 steak (ribeye, sirloin, or your favorite pork cut)
1 tsp avocado oil
1 cup fresh arugula / rocket
1 Tbsp pomegranate seeds
1 tsn fresh rosemary (optional)
Salt and pepper, to taste

Total Carbohydrates for Recipe: Approx. 6-8 grams Sugars: 3-4 grams Protein: 25-30 grams Fat: 15-20 grams Fiber: 1-2 grams Total Calories: Approx. 450-560 calories

Directions:

1. Start by taking the steak out of the refrigerator and allowing it to come to room
   temperature for about 20-30 minutes. This ensures more even cooking.

   1. While the steak is resting, preheat a stovetop grill pan or a regular skillet over medium-high heat.
   2. Brush the steak with avocado oil, then season it generously with salt and pepper on both sides.
   3. Place the steak in the hot grill pan or skillet. Cook for your desired level of doneness, about 3-4 minutes per side for medium-rare, depending on the thickness of the steak.
   4. Remove the steak from the heat and let it rest for a few minutes to allow the juices to redistribute.
   5. Meanwhile prepare the salad. In a bowl, toss the arugula with a drizzle of olive oil or mustard oil, salt and fresh cracked pepper.
   6. Arrange the arugula on a plate, top it with the sliced steak, and sprinkle the pomegranate seeds over the steak or salad.

Serve with Apple Cider Coleslaw next if desired.

Notes: It's a favorite once a week recipe being protein rich and low in carbs, making it perfect for the no sugar low carb diet.

Sesame Apple Cider Coleslaw

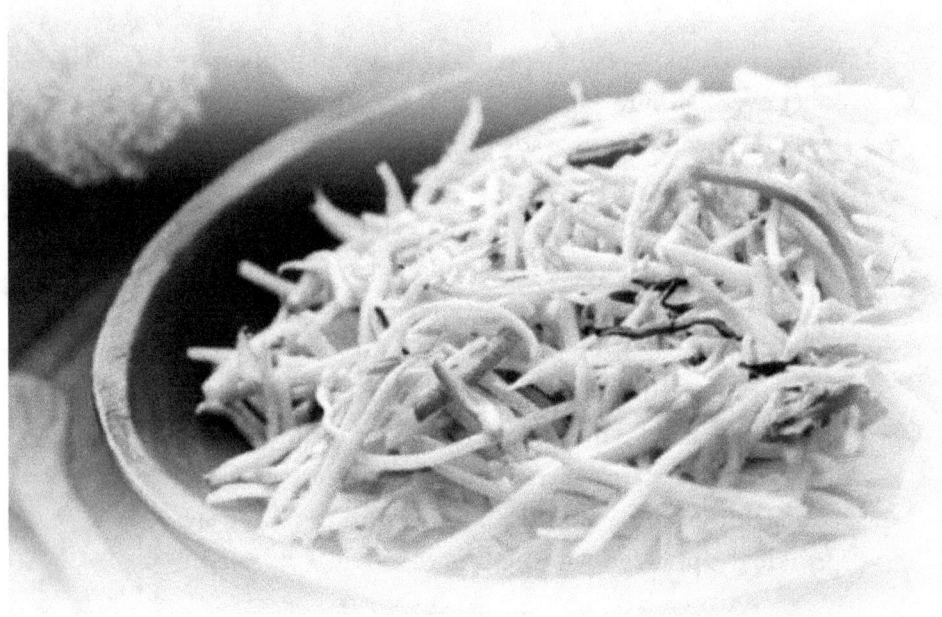

The Apple Cider Coleslaw offers a fresh and crunchy mix of vegetables with a tangy dressing. It's low in calories, provides fiber, and is a great source of vitamins and minerals.

Serving Size 1 |
Ingredients:
1 cup grated zucchini
1/2 cup grated red cabbage
1/2 carrot, grated
1 tsp olive oil
2 tsp sesame oil
1 Tbsp apple cider vinegar
1/4 tsp ground cumin (optional)
1 Tbsp of sesame and mustard seeds (optional)
Total Carbohydrates for Recipe: Approx. 12-14 grams Sugars: 6-8 grams Protein: 2-3 grams Fat: 6-7 grams Fiber: 3-4 grams Total Calories: Approx. 160-210 calories

Directions: 1. In a bowl, combine the grated zucchini, red cabbage, and grated carrot.

1. In a separate small bowl, whisk together the olive oil, sesame oil, and apple cider vinegar to create the dressing.
2. Pour dressing over the vegetables and toss well.

Notes: Goes well on the side with any fried or grilled meats. Add tofu for a change up, or add a tsp of soy sauce.

Day 6

Before Breakfast: A Glass of Water

Breakfast: Broccolini & Pepper Eggs

Lunch: Quick & Easy Chicken Salad

Dinner: Cauliflower Soup with Pan Fried Almond Fish Cakes and Oven Baked Kale Chips

Snacks: Celery or Leafy Greens

Beverages: Water, Herbal Tea or Coffee, or Fresh Ginger Tea

Nutritional Breakdown is Per Recipe (Carbs, Sugars, Protein, Fat, Fiber and Calories.) Divide by your serving size

Net Carbs = Total Carbs – Fiber

Broccolini & Pepper Eggs

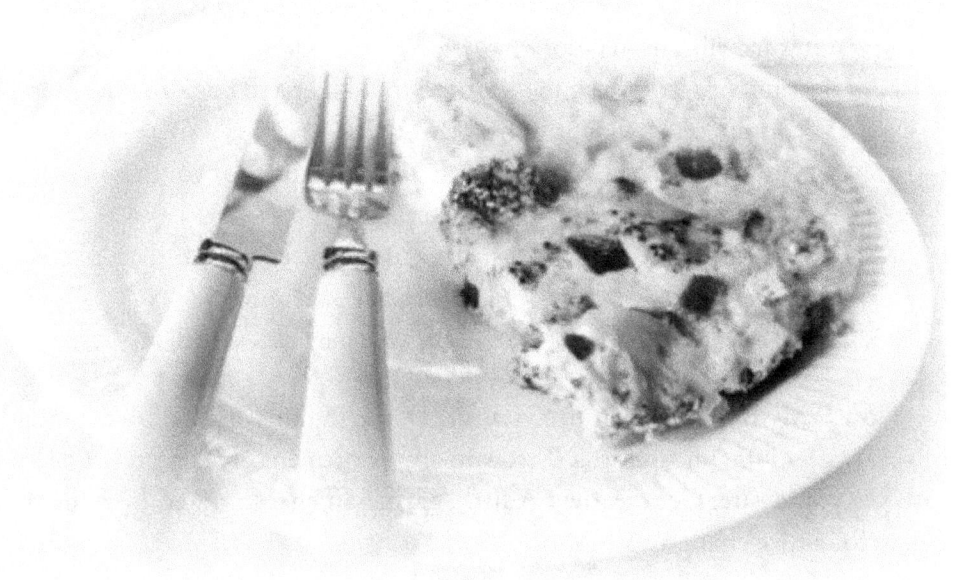

Serving Size 2 | Use leftovers with dinner or refrigerate

Ingredients:

4 eggs

1 cup chopped broccolini

1/2 cup Tofu (optional)

1 clove of garlic, diced (may use red onion)

1/4 red bell pepper, chopped (optional)

2 tsps olive oil or coconut oil

Salt, pepper, chili and spices to taste

May use leftover low carb cooked vegetables

Total Carbohydrates: Approx. 12-15 grams Sugars: 7-9 grams Protein: 30-35 grams Fat: 20-25 grams Fiber: 6-8 grams Total Calories: Approx. 440-490 calories

Directions:

1. Heat a skillet over medium-high heat and add the olive oil.

1. Add the roughly diced garlic (or finely diced red onion) to the skillet and sauté for about 1 minute until it becomes fragrant. Don't burn, it becomes bitter. Add chopped broccoli and red bell pepper to the skillet. Sauté for 3-5 minutes, or until the vegetables start to soften and turn vibrant in color.
2. If using tofu, add the cubed tofu to the skillet and cook for another 2-3 minutes, allowing it to heat through.
3. In a bowl, whisk the eggs with salt and seasonings of your choice. Pour the egg mixture into the skillet.
4. Cook, stirring gently with a spatula, until the eggs are fully cooked and scrambled, which should take about 3-5 minutes.
5. Serve for breakfast or brunch. Leftovers may be a side dish.

Notes: My hero! An egg has vitamin D, B vitamins B12, riboflavin, and minerals selenium, phosphorus. Throw in any assortment of leafy greens or low carb veg you desire. Get creative! A little parmesan cheese grated over the top makes for a nice change up.

Quick & Easy Chicken Salad

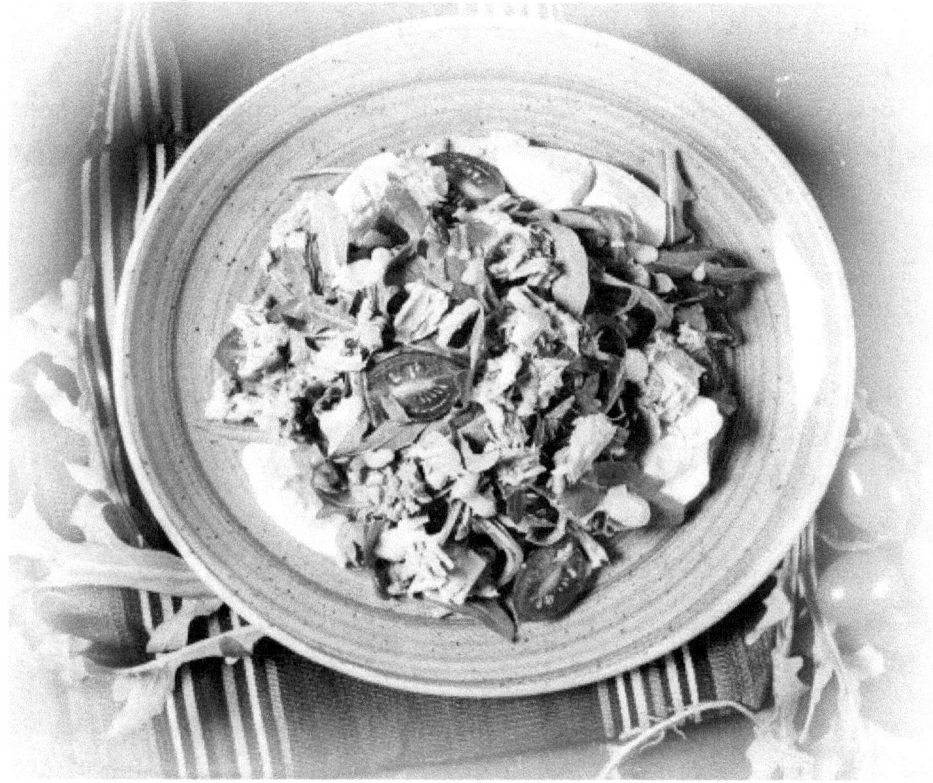

Combining protein-rich chicken, healthy fats from avocado, fiber rich chickpeas, the salad provides a well-rounded, satisfying, and nutritious meal supporting overall health and satiety.

Serving size 1-2 |

Ingredients:
1 1/2 cups cooked chicken pieces or other cold meat
2 hard- boiled eggs, halved
1 cup baby spinach leaves
1/2 cup sliced red cabbage
4 cherry tomatoes
1/4 cup chickpeas (canned and rinsed)
1 clove garlic, sliced (optional)
1/4 cup tofu or bocconcini (optional)
1 mashed avocado

Dressing:
1 tsp sesame oil
1 tsp soy sauce
1 tsp olive oil.

Total Carbohydrates for recipe: Approx. 30-35 grams Sugars: 5- 8 grams Protein: 30-35 grams Fat: 20-25 grams Fiber: 8-12 grams Total Calories: Approx. 830-890 calories

Directions:

1. In a wide salad bowl or plate, arrange the baby spinach leaves, finely sliced red cabbage, chickpeas and cooked chicken pieces.

1. If desired, add the cherry tomatoes, sliced garlic, and tofu or bocconcini to the salad.
2. Add the mashed avocado on top of the salad.
3. In a cup, whisk together the sesame oil, soy sauce, and olive oil to create the dressing.
4. Drizzle the dressing over the salad.
5. Top the salad with hard-boiled egg halves.

Notes: Great when in a hurry to get a meal together. Makes a nutritious lunch for work. The salad dressing may be omitted. I use pepitas,a generous drizzle of olive oil if not avocado. Remove chickpeas to reduce carbs.

Cauliflower Soup

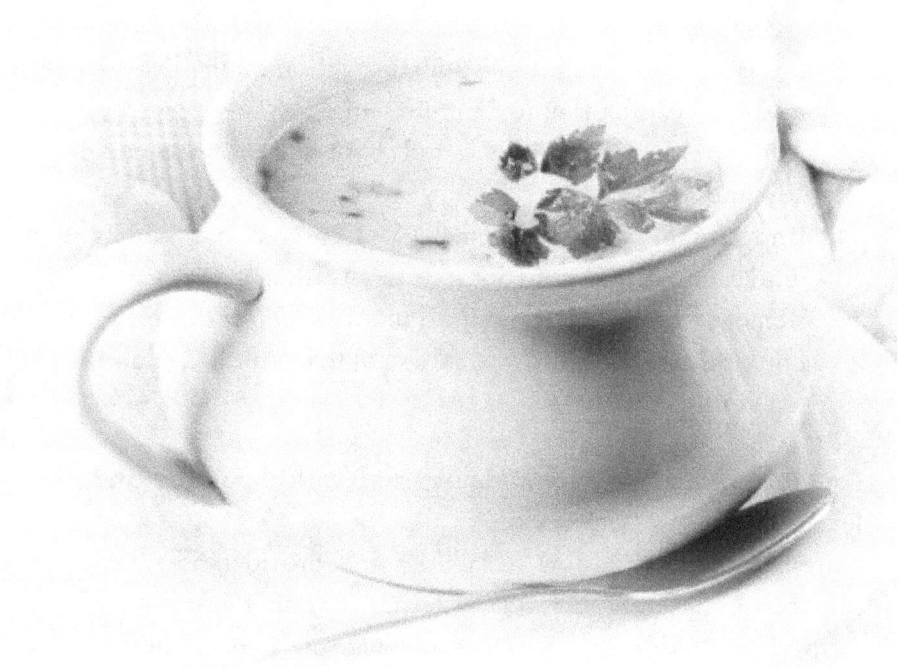

A basic, easy low carb recipe you can enjoy all year round. Refrigerate or freeze leftovers.

Serving size 2-3 |
Ingredients:
2 cups water
3 cups chicken or vegetable stock
1 head cauliflower
1 small onion
2 Tbsp olive oil (half coconut oil if you prefer a sweeter taste)
Salt and finely ground black pepper to taste
Chopped spring onion and parsley for garnish
Total Carbohydrates for recipe: Approx. 25-30 grams Sugars: 10-12 grams Protein: 5-7 grams Fat: 14-16 grams Fiber: 8-10 grams Total

Calories: Approx. 290-380 calories

Directions:

1. Clean the cauliflower of leaves and hard stems. Cut into pieces. Chop the onion.
2. In a large saucepan or stock pot saute the onion in olive oil over medium heat for around 5 minutes until soft.
3. Add the chopped cauliflower and about half the water and bring it to a simmer.
4. Bring the soup to a low simmer. Cook covered for 15-20 minutes until cauli is a little soft. Sprinkle in salt and pepper.
5. Remove from heat when done. Puree the soup with a blender wand until it is creamy. If you wish the soup to be thinner, add the remaining water.

Pour the soup in serving bowls and garnish with chopped spring onion and parsley.

Notes: Cauliflower is low in calories and provides fiber, vitamins, and antioxidants. Chicken stock adds a deeper flavour. I use homemade stock benefiting from additional nutrients and marrow rich calcium. Try adding some leftover vegetables too. If you have a benchtop blender, Multimix etc, pour soup back into the pot to reheat if necessary.

Pan Fried Almond Fish Cakes

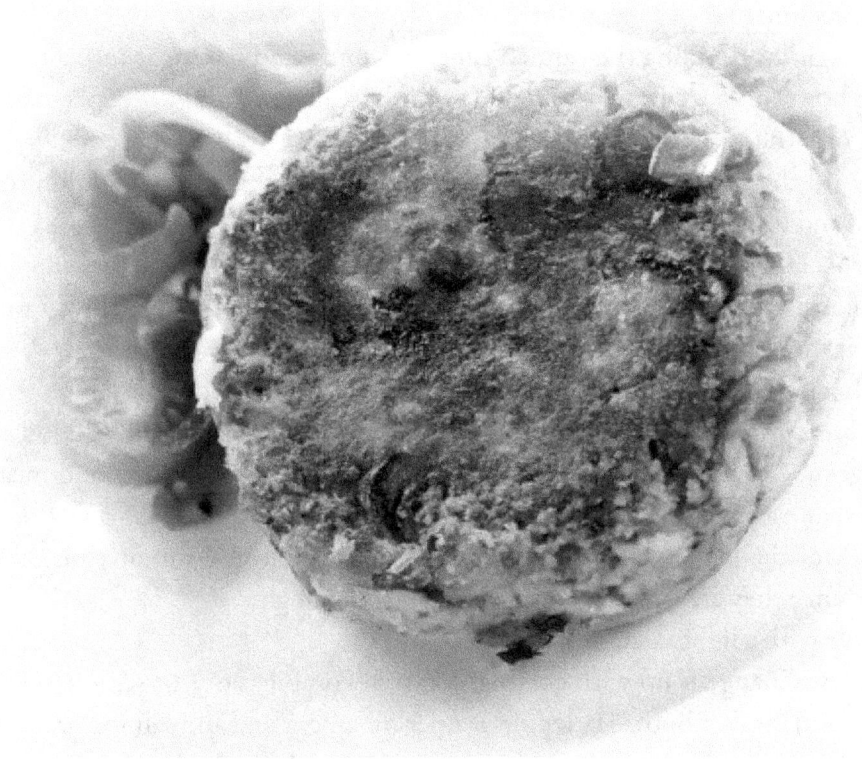

Serving size 4 | Refrigerate or freeze leftovers between greaseproof paper.
   Ingredients:
   1 Tbsp avocado oil (or half coconut oil)
   1 cup shredded zucchini
   1 egg whisked
   2 Tbsp almond meal and/or sesame seeds
   1 medium can (6oz/170g) natural tuna or salmon in olive oil drained (or use fresh steamed fish)
   1/2 cup diced green/spring onion (or chives)
   1/4 cup diced pitted olives (optional)
   1/4 tsp salt, and lemon pepper or ground black pepper
   1/4 tsp garlic or onion flakes (fresh minced is okay)

Total Carbohydrates: Approx. 15-18 grams Sugars: 2-4 grams Protein: 25-30 grams Fat: 30-35 grams Fiber: 4-6 grams

Total Calories: Approx. 500-580 calories

Directions:

1. Begin by draining the canned tuna or salmon and flaking it into a large mixing bowl. If you're using fresh steamed fish, make sure it's well-cooked and flake it into the bowl.

2. Add the shredded zucchini, whisked egg, diced green/spring onion (or chives), and diced pitted olives (if using) to the bowl.

3. Mix all the ingredients together until well combined. The mixture should have a consistency that allows you to form patties easily. If it's too wet, you can add a bit more almond meal for binding, if too dry add more egg.

4. In a separate pie dish add the almond meal/sesame seeds.

5. Heat the avocado oil in a skillet over medium heat. While the oil is heating, squeeze together Tbspns of the mixture and place into almond meal mix to shape into patties of your desired size. Set aside on a plate as you work.

5. Place the patties in the skillet and cook for about 3-4 minutes on each side, or until they are golden brown and cooked through.

Serve with a light salad or Kale chips.

Notes: Change it up with coating. I switch combinations of sesame seeds and almond meal or both. Try lemon pepper for zing. Tuna and salmon are rich in healthy omega fats. I like canned options too as they work perfectly when fresh isn't available. Use whatever fits into your lifestyle and budget.

Oven Baked Kale Chips

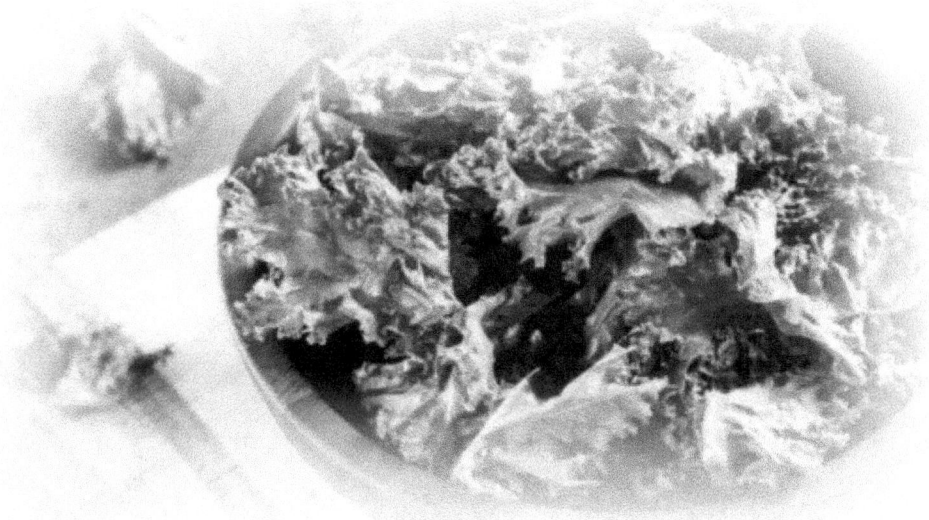

Serving size 2 | Use the same day

Ingredients:
A medium sized bunch of kale (despined)
1 tsp olive oil to drizzle
1/4 tsp salt
Total Carbohydrates: Approx. 5-7 grams
Sugars: 0-1 gram Protein: 1-3 grams Fat: 1-2 grams Fiber: 1-2 grams Total Calories: Approx. 70-90 calories

Directions:
Preheat the oven to 350°F (180°C).

1. Wash the kale and let it dry completely. Remove the hard stems and tear the leaves into large bite-size pieces. No need to use your knife. Do this by pulling down firmly along the spine beginning at wide end.
2. Sprinkle it with olive oil and salt. Toss the kale with fingers to make sure it is well coated.

3. Place kale on a baking sheet in one layer. Bake for 10 mins.

1. Once the kale is done (goes a very dark green not brown) immediately take it out of your oven and place it in a bowl or serving plate.

Notes: To prepare without using a knife simply pull down firmly along the spine starting from the wider end. Chili and onion flakes work well with this recipe. So much crunchy goodness! Kale is a nutritional powerhouse, packed with vitamins, minerals, and antioxidants. It promotes heart health, supports bone strength, and boosts the immune system. Kale is high in fiber content, aids digestion, and has anti- inflammatory properties that may reduce the risk of chronic diseases. It's a versatile and low-calorie addition to any healthy diet.

Day 7

Before Breakfast: A Glass of Water
   Breakfast: Chocolate Chia Pudding and Egg & Bacon Ramekins
   Lunch: Grilled Salmon & Pomegranate with Asparagus & Ham Salad
   Dinner: Lemongrass Beef Skewers with Easy Swiss Chard Stir Fry
   Snacks: Handful of Nuts or Leftovers
   Beverages: Water, Herbal Tea or Coffee (no sweetener or milk)

Nutritional Breakdown is Per Recipe (Carbs, Sugars, Protein, Fat, Fiber and Calories.) Divide by your serving size
Net Carbs = Total Carbs – Fiber

Chocolate Chia Pudding

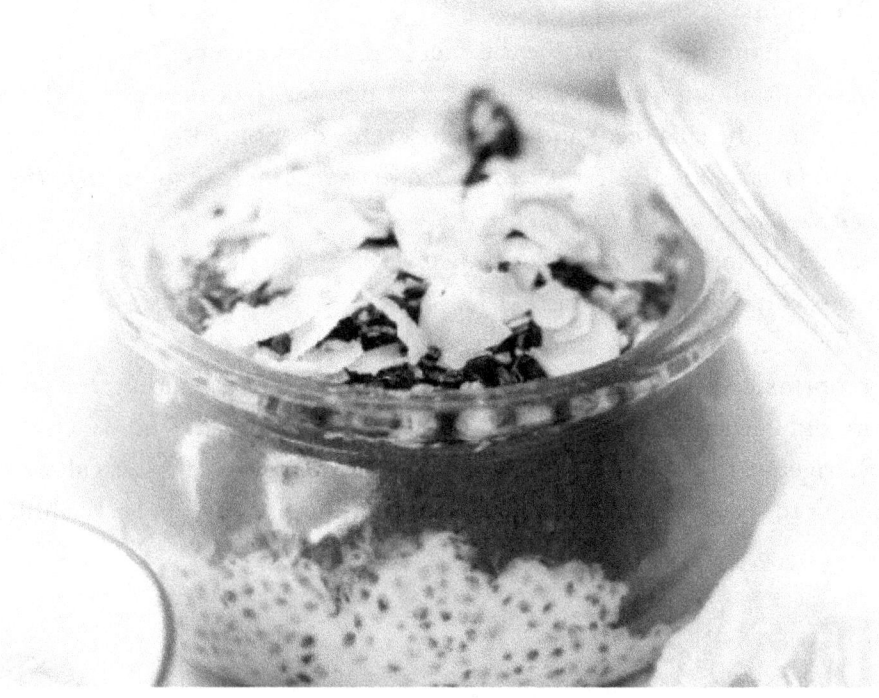

Black chia seeds are rich in fiber, omega-3 fatty acids, antioxidants, and may support heart health, weight management. You will be satiated! (This is more of a tasty dessert than pudding)

Serving size 4 | Keep sealed in the fridge, use up in 4 days or freeze into smaller pudding cups.

Ingredients:
4 Tbsp whole black chia seeds
1/4 cup heavy cream
1 cup water (or unsweetened almond milk)
1/2 Tbsp Dutch cocoa powder / raw cacao powder
2 tsp monk fruit powder
5-10 drops Stevia extract (optional)
1 tsp raw cacao nibs (or raw nuts)
A large pinch of almond flakes to garnish (optional)
Total Carbohydrates for Recipe: Approx. 20-25 grams Sugars: 2-4 grams (natural sugars and sweeteners) Protein: 5-8 grams Fat: 30-35 grams

Fiber: 10-15 grams (from chia, cocoa) Total Calories: Approx. 450-500 calories for recipe.

Directions:

1. In a mixing bowl, combine the chia seeds, heavy cream, water (or almond milk), and raw cacao powder (or cocoa powder). Mix well to ensure the chia seeds and cocoa are evenly distributed.

(Option method 2): Mix separately; cacao, stevia and 1 tsp water. Blend through the top of the pudding after step 3.)

2. Add the monk fruit powder and Stevia extract to the mixture. Adjust the sweetness and cocoa to your taste.

3. Transfer the mixture into a serving glass or jar.

4. Sprinkle the raw cocoa nibs (or raw nuts) to the pudding for added texture and flavor. Lastly add the almond flakes on top to garnish.

Refrigerate the pudding for at least a few hours, or overnight, to allow the chia seeds to absorb the liquid and create a pudding-like texture. Serve chilled.

Egg & Bacon Ramekins

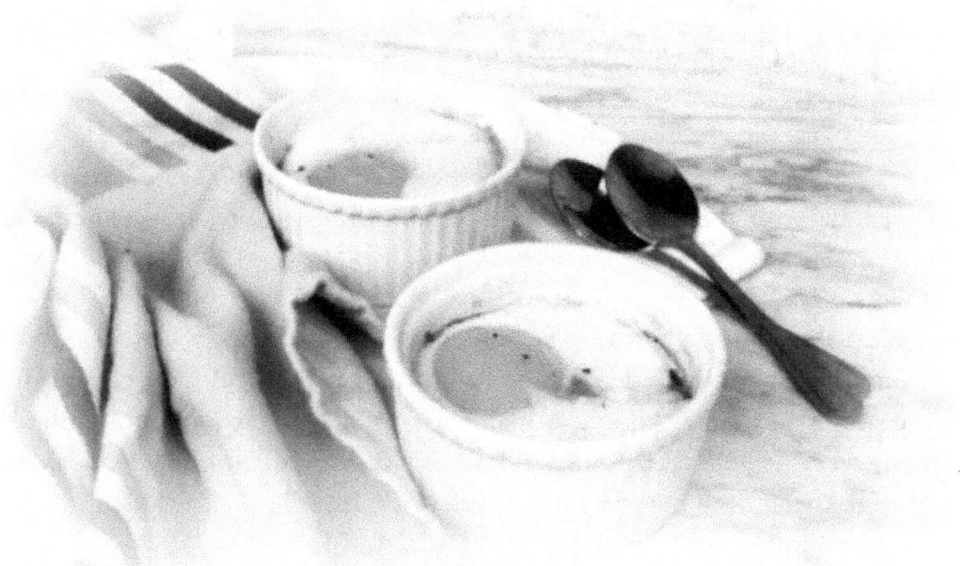

These Egg & Bacon Ramekins make for a delicious and simple breakfast or brunch dish. The eggs will be cooked with the savory flavor of the bacon or ham for a satisfying meal.

Serving Size 1-2 | Cover leftovers with plastic & refrigerate.

Ingredients:
2 tsps olive oil (to line ramekins)
2 eggs
2 rashers of bacon, turkey, spec or ham
Salt and pepper, to taste
Pinch of grated Mozzarella on top of each (optional)
Fresh or dried herbs (optional, for garnish)
Total Carbohydrates: Approx. 1-2 grams Sugars: 0-2 grams Protein: 24-30 grams Fat: 20-24 grams Fiber: Negligible Total Calories: Approx. 400-450 calories

Directions:
Preheat your oven to 350°F (175°C).

1. Lightly grease two ramekins with 1 tsp of olive oil in each to prevent sticking.
2. Line the bottom of each ramekin with a rasher of bacon or ham, creating a small nest for the eggs. You can also chop the bacon or ham into smaller pieces if preferred.
3. Carefully crack one egg into each ramekin, on top of the bacon or ham, add cheese if using, and season.
4. Place the ramekins on a baking sheet and into the preheated oven.
5. Bake for about 12-15 minutes, or until the egg whites are set and yolks are cooked as desired.

Garnish with fresh herbs. Serve hot.

Notes: Sometimes I add Mozzarella on top, and broccoli or asparagus in place of the bacon. Try adding a small amount of your favourite hot chili or onions. Very flexible with so many options! Kale chips work on the bottom rack of the oven work nicely with this dish as a side for brunch or lunch.

Grilled Salmon & Pomegranate

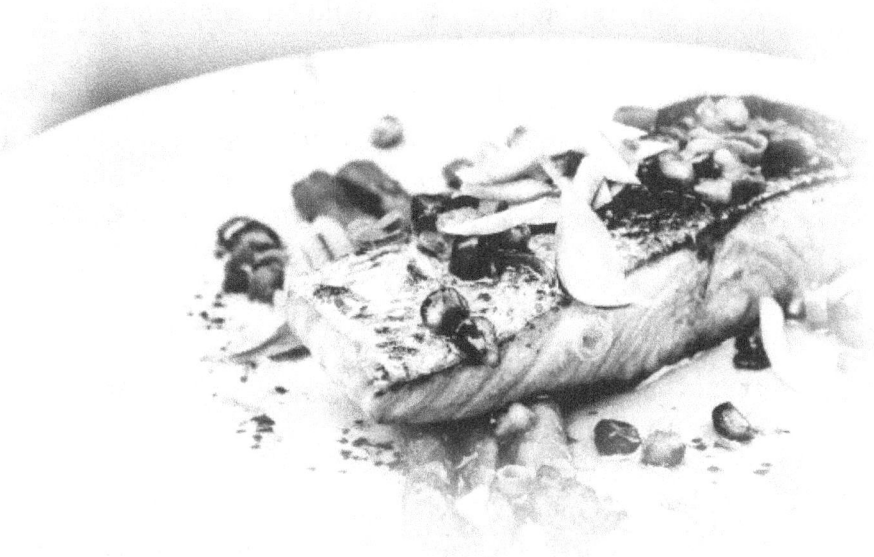

Pomegranates provide essential vitamins and minerals, such as vitamin K, potassium, and folate.

Serving size 1 | Refrigerate any leftovers.

Ingredients:
400 grams Salmon or any fresh fish (Skin off or on)
3 Asparagus spears, washed
2 Tbsp avocado oil
1/4 cup finely sliced red onion
1/4 cup pomegranate seeds for garnish
Salt and pepper to taste

Total Carbohydrates: Approx. 14-18 grams Sugars: 7-9 grams Protein: 30-35 grams Fat: 20-25 grams Fiber: 4-6 grams Total Calories: Approx. 790-880 calories

Directions:

1. Pat the salmon dry with a paper towel. Season both sides with a pinch

of salt and pepper.
2. Cook asparagus in half the oil in a skillet over medium-high heat. Cook for about 3-4 minutes, turning occasionally, until they are tender and slightly browned. Remove the asparagus from the skillet and set them aside.
3. Cook the Salmon in the same skillet, add the other Tbsp of oil. Place in the skillet, skin side down, and cook for about 4-5 minutes. Flip the salmon and continue to cook for an additional 4-5 minutes, or until the salmon is cooked to your desired firmness. The skin should be crispy, and the flesh should flake easily with a fork.
4. Arrange the cooked asparagus on a serving plate and place salmon on top, sprinkle the finely sliced red onion over the salmon and asparagus. Garnish by scattering pomegranate seeds over the dish for a burst of flavor and colour.

Notes: Pomegranates in moderation in a low-carb diet offer antioxidants, fiber, and potential heart health benefits. They're low in net carbs and versatile for adding flavor and nutrition to dishes as a garnish.

Asparagus and Ham Salad

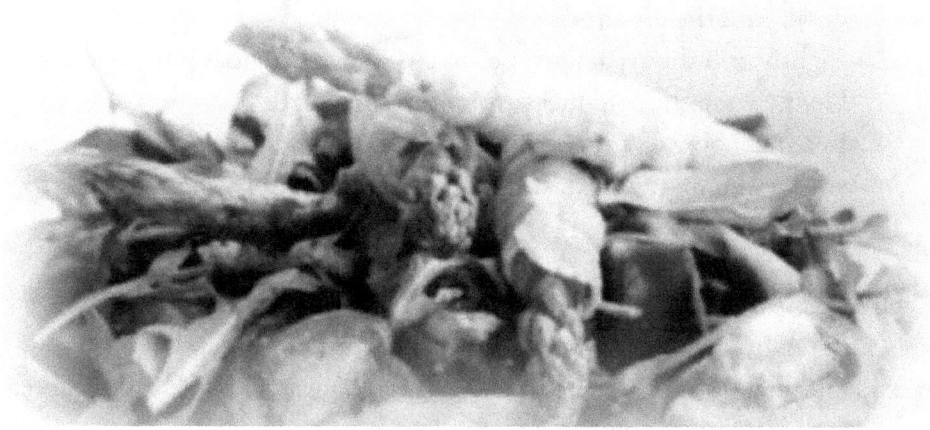

Serving size 1-2 | Good combination with Grilled Salmon

Ingredients:
4 asparagus spears, lightly grilled
2 cups arugula, rocket, or any mixed leafy green salad leaves
4 slices of fresh deli ham or other cold meat to wrap around asparagus
1 cup tomatoes, cut into big pieces
For the Vinaigrette:
2 Tbsp avocado oil
1 Tbsp apple cider vinegar
1/2 tsp Dijon mustard
Cracked pepper to taste
Total Carbohydrates: Approx. 12-15 grams
Sugars: 5-8 grams Protein: 5-20 grams Fat: 15-20 grams Fiber: 3-5 grams Total Calories: Approx. 390-450 calories

Directions:

1. Wash and dry the arugula or mixed greens, then place them in a salad bowl. Add the tomatoes.
2. Lightly grill the asparagus spears until they are tender but still crisp.
3. Gently wrap the cold meat around the asparagus
4. In a small bow or cup, whisk together the avocado oil, apple cider vinegar, Dijon mustard, and cracked pepper. Adjust the seasoning to your taste.

Drizzle the dressing over the salad ingredients.

Notes: Avocado oil is rich in monounsaturated fats and contains antioxidants, making it heart-healthy. Use any cold meat from the supermarket. The better the quality the better the overall taste.

Lemongrass Beef Skewers

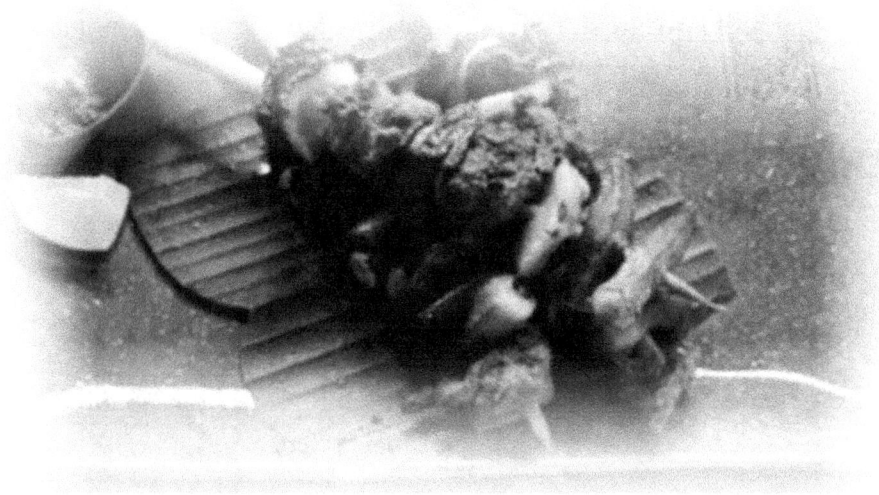

Serving size 4 | Using wooden skewers? Pre soak for 1 hr.

Ingredients:

1 pound (500 g) lean tenderloin beef, pork or chicken cut into small - medium cubes (about 1 1/2 inches)

- **2 cloves garlic, finely chopped**
- **4 lemongrass stalks (finely chopped ends)**
- **2 Tbsp natural fish sauce** (or use anchovies)
- **2 Tbsp sesame oil**
- **2 Tbsp unsweetened coconut water**
- **1 1/2 tsps ground five-spice powder**
- **1 small bunch of coriander or cilantro, finely chopped**

Total Carbohydrates: Approx. 10-12 grams Sugars: 1-3 grams Protein: 25-30 grams Fat: 12-15 grams Fiber: 2-4 grams Total Calories: Approx. 900-950 calories

Directions:

1. If using wooden skewers, soak in water for 1 hour beforehand to stop

burning.
2. Peel off the tough outer layers of the lemongrass stalks and trim the tops. You'll need the tender inner part. Then finely chop or mince.
3. Cut beef into bite size cubes to marinate meat, at least 20 minutes, but preferably overnight to intensify flavours.
4. In a bowl, mix the chopped lemongrass, garlic, fish sauce, sesame oil, coconut water, and five-spice powder.
5. Coat the beef cubes in this mixture and refrigerate for at least 30 minutes (or up to 4 hours).
6. Skewer the Beef:
7. Thread marinated beef onto skewers, leaving small gaps between pieces.
8. Grill on BBQ or stove top on a medium-high heat for 3-5 minutes per side until cooked to your personal preference.

Serve with low carb sauce, drizzle of sesame oil, or a blend.

Notes: A convenient BBQ dish that you can prepare the day before. Tender cuts work well, and even minced meat balls can be used, making this a very flexible recipe for various types of fish, pork meat etc. Simply adjust the cooking time as needed. I also enjoy using onion, zucchini, and bell pepper pieces on the skewers. If you have rosemary in the garden, tie branches together to make a basting brush, it can add great flavor. Cilantro or parsley can be used as garnish.

Easy Swiss Chard Stir Fry

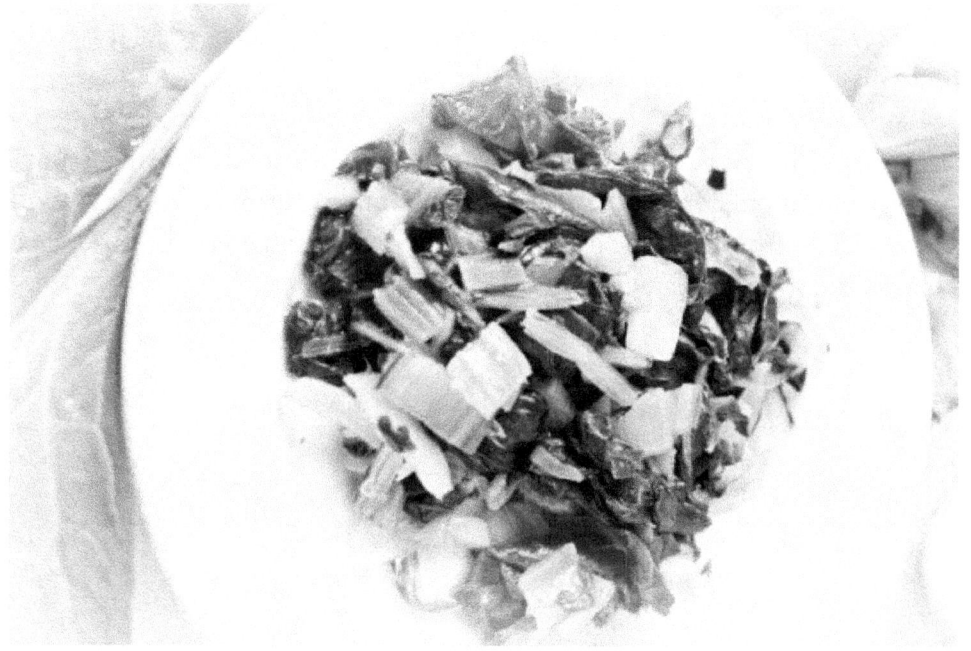

Serving size 4 | Serve with Lemongrass Beef Skewers or meat dish |
   Ingredients:
   8-10 large Swiss Chard or Silverbeet leaves, chopped
   4 garlic cloves, sliced
   3 Tbsp coconut oil
   1/2 tsp salt
   1/2 tsp of black pepper
   Total Carbohydrates: Approx. 10-12 grams
   Sugars: 1-2 grams Protein: 2-4 grams Fat: 12-15 grams Fiber: 4-6 grams Total Calories: Approx. 350-400 calories

Directions:
1. Coarsely chop the Swiss Chard leaves, roughly dice garlic cloves.
2. Heat the oil in a BBQ wok or pan, add all ingredients. Stir fry with the lid on for around 10 minutes, add a splash of water if it becomes dry. Toss a few times till tender before removing from the pan.
3. Serve with Lemongrass Beef Skewers.

Notes: The best flavored veggies are always the varieties that are in season. I grow greens throughout the year, ensuring maximum organic nutrition. Try to source locally grown organic if possible. Choose any firm green for this recipe such as Kale with spines removed

Conversion Measurement Helper

Measurement	Fluid Ounces (oz)	Milliliters (ml)	Grams (g)
1 tsp	0.17 oz	5 ml	5 g
1 tbsp	0.50 oz	15 ml	15 g
1 fl oz	1.00 oz	30 ml	30 g
1/4 cup	2.00 oz	60 ml	60 g
1/3 cup	2.67 oz	80 ml	80 g
1/2 cup	4.00 oz	120 ml	120 g
2/3 cup	5.33 oz	160 ml	160 g
3/4 cup	6.00 oz	180 ml	180 g
1 cup	8.00 oz	240 ml	240 g

Ingredient	1 cup (240 ml)	1/2 cup (120 ml)	1/4 cup (60 ml)	1 tablespoon (15 ml)
Beef	226 grams	113 grams	56 grams	14 grams
Chicken	240 grams	120 grams	60 grams	15 grams
Almond Meal	96 grams	48 grams	24 grams	6 grams
Olive Oil	216 grams	108 grams	54 grams	13.5 grams
Stock (liquid)	240 ml	120 ml	60 ml	15 ml
Raw Cocoa	80 grams	40 grams	20 grams	5 grams
Heavy Cream	240 ml	120 ml	60 ml	15 ml
Broccoli	91 grams	45.5 grams	22.75 grams	5.7 grams
Cauliflower	100 grams	50 grams	25 grams	6.25 grams
Spinach	30 grams	15 grams	7.5 grams	1.9 grams

***Measurements are approximate

Research & Resources

Special thanks to contributors; PubMed Central, American Heart Association, Nutrition Journal, Mayo Clinic, Cleveland Clinic, Google AI, USDA, WebMD.

Download Planner & Organizer from the Author

It's been a pleasure sharing, and I sincerely hope this book has guided you toward quitting sugar.

Thank you for reading :)

Peggy. NoSugarNoGrain.com

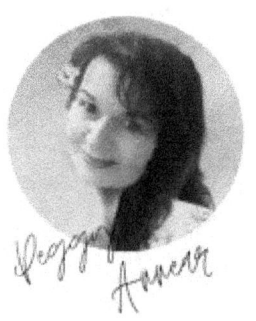

To help you organize your meals for the 7-day carb sugar detox, the meal planner will ensure that you know what's for breakfast, lunch, and dinner.

The shopping List organizer also includes a section for your goals, to do list, reminders and hydration check.

Enjoy your planner and organizer downloads next...

Printable Weekly Meal Planner

Planning ahead and writing things down before you shop can save you time, money, and reduce stress. Take Notes. Enjoy!

Scan the QR Code, Download[1] and save to your PC. Print off.

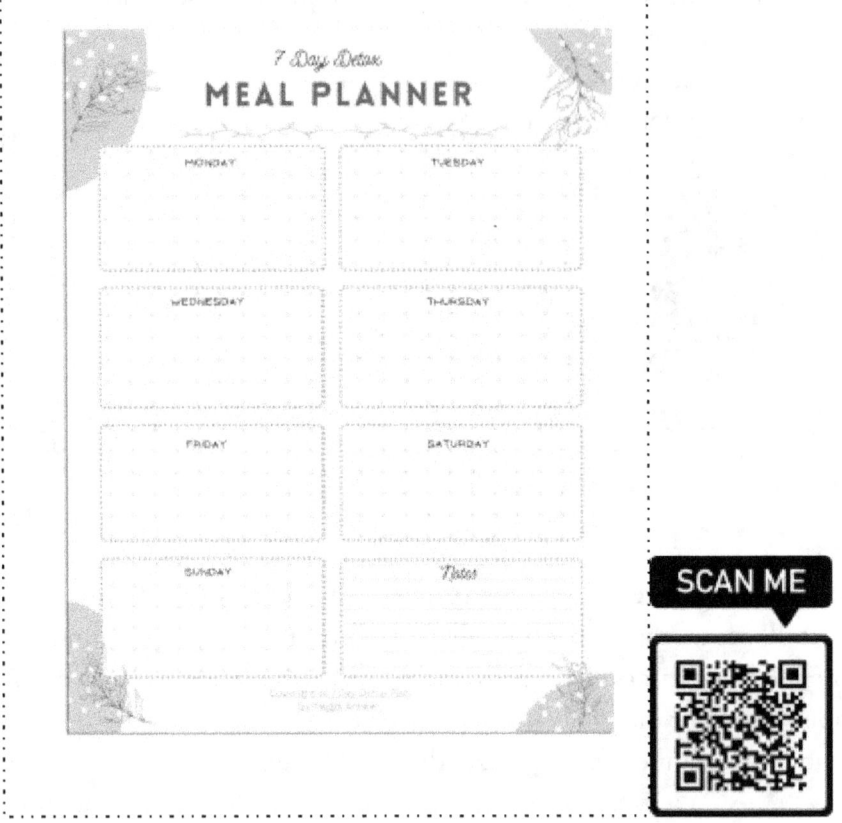

Access your Printable Weekly Meal Planner at NoSugarNoGrain.com

---

1. https://nosugarnograin.com/weekly-meal-planner-on-the-no-sugar-detox/

Bonus: A Printable Shopping List Organizer

Use it to organize your goals, shopping list, pantry...even as a reminder to drink water!

Scan the QR Code, Download[2] and save to your PC. Print off.
Printable No Sugar Shopping List Planner.

Access your Printable Shopping List Organizer at NoSugarNoGrain.com

---

2. https://nosugarnograin.com/bonus-shopping-list-planner-with-detailed-organizer/

"WATER IS LIFE'S ELIXIR, SIP BY SIP"
"KEEP YOUR EYES ON THE PRIZE, STAY FOCUSED AND ACHIEVE YOUR GOALS!

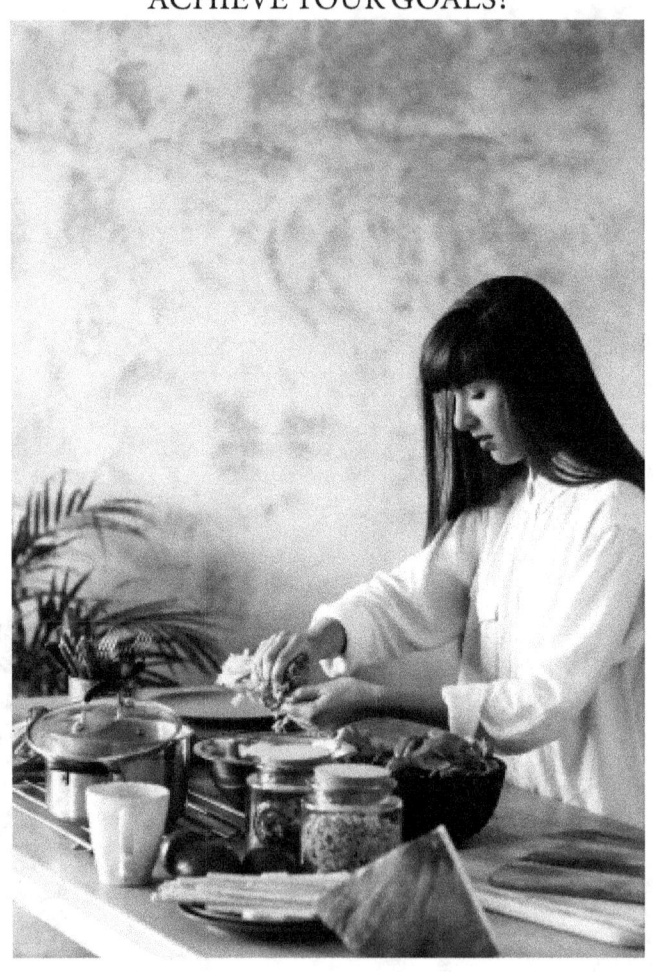

The End
...and the beginning of a new, healthier you!

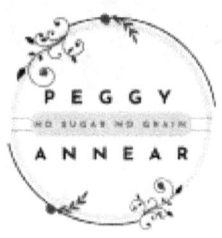

The Low Carb No Sugar Solution

The Low Carb No Sugar Solution: Copyright © 2024 by Peg E Annear

The author Peggy Annear has exclusively published this book and holds all copyrights to it. A great deal of work has been put into producing it. No part of this publication may be reproduced, stored in a retrieval system, copied in any form or by any means, electronic, mechanical, photocopying, recording or otherwise transmitted without written permission from the publisher. You must not circulate this book in any format unless asking for permission. Thank you for your honesty and understanding.

Disclaimer: This revised book encompasses extensive research and compiles nutritional information from various trusted sources, aligning with meal preparation that incorporates the principles of the no-sugar, low carbohydrate diet. It has been prepared in good faith, with the goal being to share no sugar recipe favorites and information with others. I am not liable in any way how you choose to use this information as it is an account of my own experiences. I have set out to give helpful guidance while following a no sugar low carb diet. Please consult your doctor or dietician to work out a specific plan for yourself as an individual.

www.ingramcontent.com/pod-product-compliance
Lightning Source LLC
Chambersburg PA
CBHW052140070526
44585CB00017B/1908